Gerontological Social Work Practice in Long-Term Care

The *Journal of Gerontological Social Work* series:

Gerontological Social Work Practice in Long-Term Care

George S. Getzel and M. Joanna Mellor
Editors

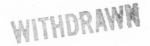

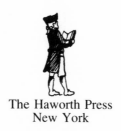

The Haworth Press
New York

Gerontological Social Work Practice in Long-Term Care has also been published as *Journal of Gerontological Social Work*, Volume 5, Numbers 1/2, Fall/Winter 1982.

The Haworth Press, Inc., 28 East 22 Street, New York, NY 10010

Library of Congress Cataloging in Publication Data
Main entry under title:

Gerontological social work practice in long-term care.

"Has also been published as volume 5, numbers 1/2 of the Journal of gerontological social work"—T.p. verso.
Includes bibliographical references.
1. Social work with the aged—Addresses, essays, lectures. 2. Aged—Care and treatment—Addresses, essays, lectures. 3. Long term care of the sick—Addresses, essays, lectures. I. Getzel, George S. II. Mellor, M. Joanna. III. Journal of gerontological social work.
HV1451.G47   1982   362.6'042   82-21371
ISBN 0-86656-146-3

Gerontological Social Work Practice in Long-Term Care

Journal of Gerontological Social Work
Volume 5, Numbers 1/2

CONTENTS

ROBERT SALMON, DSW, *Associate Dean, Hunter College School of Social Work, NY, NY,*
RENEE SOLOMON, DWS, *Associate Professor, Columbia University School of Social Work, NY, NY*
SHELDON TOBIN, PhD, *School of Social Service Administration, University of Chicago, IL*
PATTI TURENNE, *Regional Director, Hill Guthrie Association Nursing Home, Birmingham, AL*
TERESA JORDON TUZIL, MSW, *Consultant on Aging, New York, NY*
EDNA WASSER, MSW, *Consultant, Fellow, Gerontological Society, Miami, FL*
MARY WYLIE, PhD, *Professor, Department of Social Work, University of Wisconsin, Madison, WI*

ABOUT THE AUTHORS

SUSAN BLUMENFIELD, DSW, is Associate Director of the Brookdale Social Health Center for the Aging, New York, and Instructor in the Department of Community Medicine, Mount Sinai Medical Center, New York. Professional interest is in gerontological social work practice in a hospital setting.

ANN BURACK-WEISS, MSW (Social Work), is a Training Consultant at Brookdale Institute on Aging and Adult Human Development, Columbia University School of Social Work. Interests include staff development and student training in the field of gerontology. Co-author of *The Auxiliary Function Model of Social Work Practice with the Frail Elderly and their Families*, C.C. Thomas, 1982.

MARCEL O. CHARPENTIER, MSW, is Director of Social Service at the Memorial Hospital, Pawtucket, Rhode Island. Mr. Charpentier has taught at the Rhode Island College School of Social Work and is a past member of the Licensing Committee of the Rhode Island NASW chapter.

GEORGE S. GETZEL, DSW, is Associate Professor at the Hunter College School of Social Work, City University of New York, New York. As a consultant and author of several articles, Dr. Getzel's interests include group work, social work with the aged, and research in value dilemmas in working with the elderly and age identification. Dr. Getzel is a Fellow of the Gerontological Society of America.

JESSICA GETZEL, MSW (Social Work), is a Social Worker in the Department of Social Services, Jewish Home and Hospital for the Aged, New York. Ms. Getzel's interests include patient rights, reminiscence, and family policy as related to geriatric social work.

ROSE GOLDSTEIN, MSW, is Director of Social Services at the Kingsbridge Center of the Jewish Home and Hospital for the Aged, New York. Interests include work with the mentally impaired aged, Adult Day Care, and psychosocial aspects of aging.

MILDRED D. MAILICK, DSW, is Associate Professor at Hunter College School of Social Work, City University of New York. Interests include long-term care with the elderly, health care, advocacy, and collaboration as an integral part of practice. Dr. Mailick is author of numerous articles and co-editor of *Social Work in Health Services: An Academic Practice Partnership* (Prodist, 1980) and *In the Patient's Interest: Access to Hospital Care* (Prodist, in press).

M. JOANNA MELLOR, MSW (Social Work), is Trainer, Technical Assistance and Program Analyst with the Natural Supports Program of the Community Service Society, New York and an Adjunct Instructor at Fordham University, New York. Interests include the relationship of social work research to practice, the informal network of caregivers of the frail elderly, and the development of client advocacy groups.

HARRY R. MOODY, PhD, is Director of the National Policy Center on Education, Leisure and Continuing Opportunities at the National Council on the Aging, Washington, D.C. He is co-editor of the *Human Values and Aging Newsletter* and Adjunct Associate Professor of Philosophy at Hunter College, City University of New York. Interests include ethical issues in gerontology.

BARBARA JONES MORRISON, DSW, is Co-Director of the Rosenberg Center for Applied Social Work Research and Instructor in the Department of Community Medicine, Mount Sinai Medical Center, New York. Interests include socio-medical research, teaching, and ethnicity as a factor in service delivery. Dr. Morrison is involved in inter-disciplinary research on the social aspects of health and medical care and is a member of the editorial boards of *Social Work* and the *Journal of Gerontological Social Work*. Dr. Morrison is a prolific lecturer, author, and contributor to professional journals.

SUSAN N. RUBENSTEIN, MSW, is a Social Worker in the medical/ surgical inpatient service at Mount Sinai Hospital, New York where she is active within the Division of Liaison Psychiatry. Interests include work with young adult children of terminally ill parents and clinical and didactic emphasis on the psychological impact of surgery.

GARY B. SELTZER, MS (Social Work), PhD, is Assistant Professor of Community Health and Family Medicine, Brown University, and Study Director and Clinical Psychologist at Memorial Hospital, Pawtucket, Rhode Island. Interests include study of the impact of institutionalization on retarded adults, community residences, and functional assessment in primary care. He is co-author, with his wife M.M. Seltzer, of *Context for Competence: A Study of Retarded Adults Living and Working in the Community*, Cambridge Educational Projects Inc., 1978, and a contributor to several collected works.

BARBARA SILVERSTONE, DSW, is Executive Director of the Benjamin Rose Institute, Cleveland, Ohio. A past chairperson of the Committee on Aging, NASW, and of the Social Research, Planning and Practice section of the American Gerontological Society. Dr. Silverstone's interests include the aged within the family and options in long-term care. Co-author of *You and Your Aging Parent*, rev. ed. 1982 and *The Auxiliary Function Model of Social Work Practice with the Frail Elderly and their Families*, C.C. Thomas, 1982.

RENEE SOLOMON, DSW, is Associate Professor of Social Work at the Columbia University School of Social Work, New York. Interests include services to the elderly, social work practice with old people and their families, staff development and training. Dr. Solomon acts as consultant to psychiatric and geriatric hospitals and is author of numerous articles.

MARILYN E. WILSON, MSW, is Grant Associate of the Hunter College School of Social Work, City University of New York, Instructor in the Department of Community Medicine at the Mount Sinai School of Medicine consortium. Interests include social work teaching within a health care setting.

ANNA H. ZIMMER, MSW, is Director of the Natural Supports Program, Community Service Society, New York and a member of the Advisory Committee of the National Council of Jewish Women, Brooklyn Section. Interests include family counseling and social policy issues as related to the informal support network of the frail elderly.

FOREWORD

This is one of the first two volumes in our Social Work Practice Series published by The Haworth Press.

George S. Getzel and M. Joanna Mellor have done an excellent job, both in the introductory chapter which they wrote and in their selection of authors and content areas. Some of the articles, the Jessica Getzel piece on Residents Council (Ch. 11), Renee Solomon's on Serving Families (Ch. 4), Chapter 7 on Sociocultural Dimensions by Barbara Jones Morrison, and Harry R. Moody's article on Ethical Dilemmas (Ch. 5), for example, are specific to the institutional settings. Others are written from the perspective of the acute treatment hospital social worker, the social worker in the community, the social worker in a rehabilitation center.

Properly, I think, all of the authors imbed their work in particular service settings; properly because it is the nature of social work practice that the worker-client relationship is never in a social vacuum. The agency or institution is not only the setting for the relationship; it is also part of the calculus, and similarly our definition of the client is always one which contains both person and situation. The emphasis, therefore, on setting is necessary in each chapter, but that is not to say that the nature of this volume and the individual pieces are limited to social workers in these settings.

The Morrison article, for example, should be of interest to administrators and practitioners in area agencies, senior centers and other community service agencies as well as to the staffs of Long-Term Care Facilities, and her "Suggested Guidelines for Practice" merit particularly careful study. In a like fashion, although Moody deals with ethical dilemmas which are characteristic in the institutional setting, they are not unique to this setting. His "Taxonomy of Ethical Issues," the distinction he makes between "Ethical Dilemma and Practical Problem," and his thoughtful discussion of "Ethical Theories" offer valuable approaches for all who work in the field of aging—regardless of profession or setting.

The Silverstone and Burack-Weiss chapter on the Social Work Function and Solomon's on Work with Families should be read sequentially, I think. Silverstone and Burack-Weiss make a strong case, on both conceptual and pragmatic grounds, for thinking of the Social Work Function in Long-Term Care in a way which gets us past the distinction between the institutional and community setting. The focus here is on the characteristics of the aged population whose health status makes long-term care necessary. Such a focus then permits more systematic attention to service needs, professional function, and social work practice.

Solomon narrows the range to examine in-depth the four crises in the career of the old person and family if placement in an institution becomes necessary. Again, although the article is setting specific, there is much practice wisdom that should be of general usefulness.

I have selected these articles for special mention, but not with any implication of selectivity based on excellence. Every chapter of this volume is worthy of careful reading: the selection was designed simply to illustrate the range of topics.

Professionals in the field will be indebted to Getzel and Mellor for this volume. It is truly *must* reading.

Rose Dobrof

Gerontological Social Work Practice in Long-Term Care

INTRODUCTION: OVERVIEW OF GERONTOLOGICAL SOCIAL WORK IN LONG-TERM CARE

Long-term care provision for the aged is rapidly becoming a preeminent concern of society. The accelerating proportion of older persons living longer results in expanding needs for health and social services and income maintenance benefits. This volume explores the changing functions and roles of professional social workers serving the elderly, their families and other support systems.

We view long-term care as defined by Elaine Brody to include nursing homes and community services.[1] As repeatedly documented in social gerontological research, kin, friends and neighbors provide the preponderance of long-term care to the moderately and severely impaired elderly in the community.[2] It appears that research on family caregiving is beginning to make a major impact on service design and the way in which social workers in direct service intervene with older persons and their networks. Work with kin and other persons who form informal helping networks is becoming a primary element of the emerging practice framework for gerontological social work.

The social worker's historical concern with human beings at the point of interface with the environment has special utility for work with the elderly. The environment that fits the changing needs of older persons contributes to their enhanced autonomy, competence and self-esteem. A biopsychosocial conception of human beings is crucial in helping the aged. Assessment for social work intervention with and on behalf of the elderly involves a sophisticated understanding of lifelong development, human aging and those particular health, social and economic conditions that individually and cumulatively challenge the elderly's adaptive and creative capacities.

Social workers must be knowledgeable and sympathetic to the growing numbers of functionally impaired elderly in our midst. Our ageist society with its adulation of youth and cosmetic solutions to aging makes the job of class and case advocacy difficult. Social workers will be called on not only to help the elderly, but also to interpret the scope and mean-

1

ing of aging to a society which has little experience with a "graying" population.

The social worker's educative function on behalf of the interests and well-being of the elderly arises out of the service situation and the ontological questions about human aging. Gerontological social work practice is inextricably tied to interprofessional collaboration. The social worker's concern with the psychosocial well-being of individuals, groups and families develops in the context and as a consequence of the actions of nurses, administrators, physicians, psychologists, occupational therapists, nursing aides, and others. Social workers must acquire substantive knowledge of other professional orientations and the theoretical and practice concepts that influence how these professionals work with older persons. Human aging is a persistent and demanding encounter with human finitude. Ernest Becker writes that "Man wants to know that his life has somehow counted, if not for himself, then at least in a larger scheme of things, that it has left a trace, a trace that has meaning."[3] To the extent that we conceive of aging as emblematic of the end of life, practitioners face continuing emotional and value dilemmas. To the extent to which the aged are viewed as damaged objects, symbols of our own frailty, we seek impersonal solutions. Given the "cost" of long-term care, conveniently cast into dollars and cents, we may ask whether long-term care is necessary, unlimited, right or good? Should heroic lifesaving technology be applied to the old and to what extent should the wishes of families or old persons themselves determine the interventions used and the care provided? Social workers, as well as other professionals, struggle with difficult value questions which hold direct implications for ethical conduct.

This book is not an exhaustive survey of what social workers need to know or do. Frankly, at this time such a task is beyond any one book. The primary emphasis is an examination of direct practice grounded in immediate program and policy context. We commend works by Brody,[4] Lowy[5] and Brearley[6] which have attempted a systematic discussion of social work in long-term care, and aging and social work respectively. It is urgent that social workers keep up to date with gerontological research findings in the social and behavioral sciences, medicine, biology and policy analysis. We may be approaching the time when gerontological social workers will develop subspecialities according to the setting (acute care, rehabilitation, home care) and/or the target population (families, aging couples, diabetic older patients).

In an effort to plant service aspirations firmly in the realities of practice, contributors represent both "town and gown," practitioners and aca-demics. Most chapters contain actual examples from practice to illustrate the flow of process that corresponds to practice principles. No effort has been made to fit the perspectives of contributors into a neat package. Where perspectives clash, readers are encouraged to choose sides based on their own value stances and experiences.

In the first section, Barbara Silversone and Ann Burack-Weiss make the case for a model of social work practice which is at once broad yet informative and that describes the multidimensional levels of actions open to skilled professionals in home care and in nursing home settings. Susan Blumenfield looks at the medical center as a key location for the care of the elderly during acute episodes. Assessment of the elderly, collabora-tion and education of staff become major tasks. Gary Seltzer and Marcel Charpentier look imaginatively at rehabilitation centers as an integral part of the continuum of care for the frail elderly. Tools for assessment and modes of intervention in collaboration with other professionals are discussed.

In the second section, Renee Solomon illuminates four crises faced by family members concerning their frail institutionalized relatives and sug-gests differential intervention strategies. Harry Moody provokes us with the question, "Why provide long-term care to the elderly?" He clearly and succinctly describes a range of value dilemmas that belie many prac-tice issues. Mildred Mailick examines aging and illness as interactive process. She proposes a conceptual formulation and suggests its utility to the practitioner. Barbara Morrison looks at minority elderly in nursing homes. She specifies their unique needs, patterns of adaptation and family linkages which have significant implications for practice and program development.

The final section consists of practice innovations and issues identified and analyzed by practitioners in hospitals, nursing homes, home care and family support programs.

We hope this volume will stimulate an interest and renewed commit-ment to service by student social workers and veteran practitioners alike. In an excellent historical review of social work and aging, Louis Lowy writes "it is now recognized that this significant client and target popula-tion has a right to quality services and that practice with the aging will affect the whole of social work practice in the immediate and long-range future."[7] In the current period of contracting resources diverted into military expenditures, the social worker's commitment to the aged will be tested even more rigorously. The younger generations may be goaded into making claims for resources at the expense of the old. It is therefore imperative that social workers strive to maintain high standards of service and to monitor the quality of these services and the elderly's well-being so as to be able to advocate on their behalf with factual precision and passion in these dark days.

George S. Getzel
M. Joanna Mellor

REFERENCES

1. Brody Elaine L. *Long-Term Care of Older People: A Practical Guide*. New York: Human Sciences Press, 1977.

2. General Accounting Office. "Home Care for a National Policy to Better Provide for the Elderly." HRD 78-L9, Washington, D.C., December 30, 1977, and Ethel Shanas, "The Family as a Social Support System in Old Age," *Gerontologist, 19*, April 1979, pp. 169-740.

3. Becker, Ernest. *Escape from Evil*. New York: Free Press, 1975, p. 4.

4. Brody, *op. cit.*

5. Lowy, Louis. *Social Work With the Aging: The Challenge and Promise of Later Years*. New York: Harper and Row, 1979.

6. Brearley, C.P. *Social Work, Aging and Society*. London & Boston: Routledge and Kegan, Paul.

7. Lowy, *op. cit.*, p. 19.

Part I

SETTINGS FOR PRACTICE

Chapter 1

THE SOCIAL WORK FUNCTION
IN NURSING HOMES AND HOME CARE

Barbara Silverstone
Ann Burack-Weiss

Until recently, social work functions in nursing homes and in home care programs were regarded as rather separate fields of practice, with disparate goals and different types of clients. In the nursing home setting, the social worker's central task was to facilitate the adjustment of the client to the institution. In community home care settings, the social worker's central task was to foster to the extent possible independent functioning on the part of the client. Nursing home clients were viewed as permanently dependent, either for physical, mental, social, and/or emotional reasons, and in need of long-term care. Community home care clients were viewed as much more in control of their lives, with a need for short-term or occasional services to support them in crisis situations.

Social work practice in these settings has closely paralleled changes in the concept of long-term care which in the past was equated with nursing home placement. Now it is viewed as encompassing both institutional and community services. The burgeoning number of very old people in our society has contributed to this view, and the startling fact that for very old, frail, or impaired older persons living in nursing homes, there are counterparts living in the community. What seems to differentiate these populations is not so much the level of disability, but the fact that older people in nursing homes are poorer and more socially isolated.[1] Family caregiving, comprising 80% of the total care given to the elderly, appears to be the most important factor in avoiding and deterring institutionalization, although there is growing evidence that families are greatly

This chapter is adapted from the authors' text—*The Auxiliary Function Model of Social Work Practice with the Frail Elderly and their Families*, to be published by C.C. Thomas, the book is scheduled for release in late 1982.

7

burdened.[2] All in all, disillusionment with the quality and expense of institutional care, a growing awareness that many frail and disabled elderly can remain in the community with less costly support, and an increasing consumer demand on the part of the old and their families for community-based care have sparked a modest increase in these services to the frail elderly.

A view of long-term care which bridges community and institutional settings is receiving further validation from experts in the field who recognize the fluctuating and complex needs of the chronically impaired client who might profit from care in both settings, either simultaneously or consecutively. Institutionally based day care, while not widespread, is cited as an excellent intervention for some frail elderly and as a respite for family members. Short-term use of nursing home beds at times of crisis or for family respite is being considered as well as congregate housing with strong support services for the physically frail.[3]

These developments in long-term care—the pragmatic and the conceptual—offer compelling reasons for a shift in social work practice from one in which goals are defined by the specific nature of the setting (which presumably serves a particular type of client) to goals which are defined by the problem and the needs of the frail, impaired client wherever he is encountered along the continuum of care. The very fact that the settings of nursing home and community home care can serve clients with similar problems and needs makes this argument all the more compelling. This is also in the mainstream of current social work practice in which interventive modalities and the worker's role are seen as dictated by salient aspects of the client's problem rather than predetermined by the preference or policy of the helping agency. Yet it still must be recognized that the unique organizational characteristics of institutional and community settings require special practice approaches.

This chapter will examine the commonalities in social work practice in community home care and institutional settings and the unique aspects of practice in each setting. Other important settings along the continuum of long-term care, particularly the hospital and day care, will be discussed in other chapters. First, an overview of the problems and needs of the client population is in order.

Problems and Needs of the Frail and Impaired Elderly and their Families

The elderly population, a large and diversified one spanning a number of generations, is being increasingly referred to as the young-old and the old-old with 65-75 and over 75 as the arbitrary cutoff points. It is the old-old population who are generally referred to as frail, an accepted euphemism for the marked acceleration of the aging process and the incidents of disease in this age group. There are, of course, those under 75, and even 65, who would be considered frail and those over 75 who are not. The important point to note here is that frailty is not a ubiquitous gerontological condition but prevalent enough to warrant the most serious consideration. Current estimates of functional disability in the over 65 population are as high as 17%.[4]

There appears to be general consensus in the health and social service field that the key problem facing the frail, impaired person is not of disease or old age but the effects these conditions have on mental and physical functioning, particularly in relation to the activities of daily living: housekeeping, cooking, bathing, dressing, toileting, shopping, chores, and money management. The inability to function in one or more of these areas creates some degree of dependency on others for the performance of these tasks, more often than not on the family. Senile Alzheimer's Disease, cardiovascular conditions, arthritis, osteoporosis, and sensory impairments are probably the most crippling of diseases.[5]

While the level of mental and physical functioning is viewed as a more important measure of the frail elderly's needs for long-term care than the medical diagnosis, the latter is important in determining the etiology of a functional impairment. All too often diseases and ensuing functional impairments are viewed as the irreversible and inevitable consequences of old age. In some cases, careful investigation reveals reversible conditions such as malnutrition or drug toxicity which can be ameliorated.

The level of functioning, in terms of the measured ability to perform certain tasks, falls far short of identifying the problems and needs of the frail elderly. Functioning must be placed within a broader psychological and ecological context. Just as the underlying physical condition effects functioning, so do these other factors, which can include a wide range of environmental and personal conditions: poverty, housing and transportation barriers, lack of social supports, depression, anxiety, and excessive psychosocial dependence among others. If one or more of these factors, singly or in combination, interfere with functioning, they can constitute a serious cluster of problems for a frail elderly person. Their effects can be rebounding and cumulative, calling for a multifaceted approach to meeting the elder's needs.

> Mrs. J., 80 years of age, widowed with no close relatives, had been stricken with arthritis of the hip which prevented her from

shopping for herself particularly since she lived in a second-floor walk-up. Her hands were also afflicted, and she was unable to cook with traditional equipment. Her poor nutrition only exacerbated the mild confusion she had been experiencing and the depression she has suffered since the death of her husband. These latter conditions contributed further to her difficulty in coping with the tasks of daily living.

Elderly neighbors, who had been attempting to meet some of her needs, had referred Mrs. J. for help. Special transportation and services in the home were needed to sustain Mrs. J. in the community if only to provide her with adequate nutrition. Health care services were required to address her physical and mental symptoms as well as increased social contacts to compensate for the loss of husband and friends. But first, someone was needed to establish contact with Mrs. J. and to provide the crucial human links to help and services which had been missing in her life since her husband's death.

A critical aspect of the frail older person's situation is the depleting effects of frailty itself as well as a host of other losses. There are indeed older people who bounce back after crises or compensate in some way for their losses. But for the very old person in particular the effects of the aging process itself must be considered: the slowing down, the heightened sensory thresholds which diminish input from the environment, the weakening of intrasystemic boundaries which undermine resiliency. The individual's coping capacities can be adversely affected as a direct result of decline and illness. Regardless, of the degree of person-environment fit achieved, internal developmental processes are underway which make the frail elder highly vulnerable and require a strategic approach specifically designed to counteract the effects of depletion and loss.

The auxiliary function defines this individualized approach. It is a loan transaction in which the impaired client borrows what is needed for as long as it is needed. The goal is conservative: to replenish resources that have proven functional for the client throughout life in the belief that innate drives toward mastery and optimum adaptation can prevail, given a prosthetic boost.

Relationship with a significant other is the medium through which the auxiliary function is provided. This emotional bond and attachment with a constant caring figure is as crucial at the end of life as at the beginning. The sense of worth and self-esteem, eroded by failing powers and a dependent state, is buttressed by the concern and borrowed strength of another. The auxiliary function may overlap or be distinct from physical caretaking functions. It is most commonly carried out by the family who also provides the great bulk of care to the frail elderly and whom the elderly usually turn to at times of crisis. The social worker may perform the auxiliary function, share it with other members of the helping team, or assist family members in assuming the role. Who fills the role is less important than the fact that affective as well as instrumental needs of the frail older client are addressed.

The Commonalities in Social Work Practice:
The Auxiliary Function Model

To whatever the extent the auxiliary function is assumed by the social worker, it is a concept which undergirds our work with the frail elderly and defines the commonalities of practice in the nursing home and home care setting. The auxiliary function contains several elements which in combination can be viewed as a model. These functional elements include a supportive relationship and the carrying out of interpreting, mediating, advocacy, and monitoring transactions. The affective aspects of the function are as important as, and are often a prelude to, instrumental ones. Feelings of helplessness in the face of multiple losses may be ameliorated by an emotional bonding with a stronger and/or empathic other who conveys a sense of hope.[6] When carried out directly or indirectly by the social worker, the auxiliary function adheres to the principles of client self-determination in that his intent as dictated by present wishes and past life-styles are adhered to.

An ecological and developmental approach which addresses the wide spectrum of factors impinging on the elderly underlies practice commonalities in nursing home and home care and the use of the auxiliary function model. The study, assessment, and plan; direct practice with client or clients and family systems; and community and service systems interventions provide a traditional and useful framework for discussing of practice similarities. Practice differences as determined by each setting are then examined.

The Study, Assessment, and Plan

A *study* and *assessment* of a frail elder's problems are an undertaking more complex than for younger persons. Not only has the older client brought to old age the accumulated experiences of a lifetime which influence his present behavior, but current functional problems and other closely related ones susceptible to rapid intersystemic changes. The study and assessment are separate but overlapping processes. The study refers to the collection of information about the client, family, and their situation. The assessment is the worker's interpretation of this accumulated information: the location, cause, interrelationship, and prioritization of the problems. It is important that the assessment be articulated by the worker and summarized in writing and shared with the clients as it then becomes an explicit raison d'être for *the plan* open to modification and changes as the client's situation changes. In fact, the *study* and *assessment* are an important intervention in and of themselves, since clients and families come to know and understand their situation better through the process. Sorting out of problems for the frail client can be an important auxiliary intervention and, if necessary, a time when a strong worker-client alliance is established.

The order of the information that should be gathered as the study proceeds should follow the direction of client and family. No rigid structure should be imposed, lest valuable information be lost. If the family or older person seems ready and eager to talk about the past, the social worker can grasp the opportunity for insight into habitual coping patterns. If the family or older person are most eager to talk about the here and now, current efforts to meet their needs can be explored. Functional assessment schedules which social workers may utilize should be used as supplements to the interviewing process, not as a guiding tool. The client must be met where he or she is, a clear understanding reached for the work to be undertaken together, and beginning trust established if accurate information is to be gathered.

> 80-year-old, blind Mr. G., who had been referred by friends for home and health aide services, was reticent to discuss his functioning problems with the social worker. There were a number of pictures on the wall of him as a younger man fishing in different parts of the world. He eagerly responded to the worker's interest in this former activity and after a while could share with her his present plight.

Ecosystems and development perspectives serve as the organizing framework for the information gathered in the study and for the formulation of the assessment. An ecosystems perspective provides an adaptive view of human beings in constant interchange with all elements of their environment.[7] A developmental perspective views individual and family adaptation over the life cycle.[8] The concept of the auxiliary function, however, must serve as the fulcrum on which all other information about the client and his situation is balanced, that is to say, in what areas is he now dependent for help and who can best provide it.

The assessment of frailty should be an interdisciplinary judgment based upon the functional assessment, medical diagnosis, and age of the client. A mistaken judgment about frailty, of course, can always be corrected in an assessment process open to change.

The network of social supports, formal and informal, surrounding the client are identified and described. What is the capacity for performing the auxiliary function and for providing practical support such as chore services? What is the meaning of these supports to the older person in addition to caregiving? What are the transactions between the client and these helping or potentially helping systems? The physical environment must be described in terms of the barriers it presents to the client and the client's coping capacities in relation to these barriers. If the family plays an important auxiliary role, then problem-solving capacities should be specified.

At some phase of the study and assessment a look at the past is in order. Links between now and then frequently arise spontaneously in initial interviews. Families and older people can change over the life cycle—sometimes dramatically—but they often resort to coping mechanisms which served them in the past and which is built upon by the auxiliary function.

More obvious social factors which need to be elicited are the interests, pleasures, and habits of old persons over their life span. This information is particularly important for nursing home personnel who wish to provide recreation and other social inputs, but also in planning for persons remaining in their own homes whose social sphere has been severely constricted and lifelong pleasures diminished. For even the most disabled there must be some replenishment of these activities if their daily lives are to be worth the effort of survival.

The plan should never be decided upon and enacted until an assessment has been made, i.e., when the worker believes there is enough information about and understanding of a problem to know what should be done. By the same token, a *plan* should not be delayed because the worker must first collect an overabundance of information irrelevant to the situation at hand. In emergency situations, when temporary plans must be made, caution directs that these not be irrevocable.

The formulation of *the plan* should be a collaborative endeavor between client and worker. In the case of an involved family it is part of a group problem-solving process. If the worker is to fill the auxiliary function role, it is a step forward in what is hopefully a productive worker-client relationship. The worker should guard against being coerced by time pressures or the anxiety of client, family members, and others to move precipitously. Side taking with one family member, the whole family, or the elder should be avoided. The plan involves specific long- and short-term goals. The means of achieving these goals will involve the elder and others.

Disability and frailty do not preempt the possibility of functional improvements on the part of the elder even if they are minimal. The challenge implicit in goal setting can offset the regressive tendencies which can affect the depleted client. Short- and long-term goals also serve as stimuli to the helping team to measure and evaluate their own therapeutic inputs which they may tend to diminish in work with the very old. If the auxiliary function role does not require the skills of a professional social worker, a short-range goal may be to transfer this role.

> Long-term home health aide services were planned with Mrs. S., an 85-year-old widow, who was depressed and functioning poorly in a number of areas. Her severe arthritis accounted for some of this malfunctioning. The assessment suggested that a good bit of this malfunctioning was owing to the lingering depression she had suffered since her husband's death 2 years ago.
>
> A plan was agreed upon with Mrs. S. to provide long-term home-maker services to her, yet with the expectation that the number of hours could be decreased as short-term goals were reached. The first short-range goal was to help her to come to grips with her widowed role and to explore other social resources. The second short-range goal was to learn a series of skills at home to compensate for her arthritis. The long-range goal was to reduce visits from the home health aide from five to two visits a week and to help a concerned and friendly neighbor to share the auxiliary role.

Direct Practice with the Client

The extent of social work involvement with a frail client will depend on a number of factors. Foremost is the availability of others to perform the auxiliary function. When the actual frailty and impairment of the client have been determined and there is no one willing or able to fill this role, it is imperative that the social worker assume this responsibility. A trusting relationship, the very cornerstone of the auxiliary function role of the social worker may arise spontaneously in the course of shared activity. More often it is fostered through a variety of techniques and skills which tangibly illustrate the worker's respect and concern, competence and reliability.

Consideration must first be given to the role of the client whose very frailty and impairments may discourage the worker from observing the customs commonly adhered to in adult transactions. Conscious efforts may be required on the part of the worker with the frail client, particularly if the elder feels his role is a diminished one and behaves in an obsequious manner. The setting of appointment times is an important first step.

> Since the worker knew Mrs. J. would be home at any time because of her severe arthritis and inability to travel, he decided to drop in sometime during the week to complete the application process. The worker telephoned 15 minutes in advance when he found he was in Mrs. J.'s neighborhood. The client discounted his having inconvenienced her, but throughout the interview was quite distraught and suspicious. This behavior was viewed by the worker as being symptomatic of mental impairment on Mrs. J.'s part, rather than as a result of his intrusiveness.

The setting of an appointment time at least 24 hours in advance (in institution, office, as well as home settings), immediately conveys the worker's expectation in relation to the client's adult role—a participating active one. It gives the elder the opportunity to prepare for the interview and to feel and actually be more in control of his or her situation.

The interview setting should be carefully prepared, be it in the client's home, the worker's office, or the client's bedside. As much privacy as possible should be sought and distracting noises minimized. Given the sensory deficits common to old age, arrangements should be made for the worker to be able to directly face the client, speaking slowly and distinctly. The presence of others, such as family or friends, should be at the discretion of the elder—at least for some interviews.

The older client should be addressed by his last name in spite of the client's apparent willingness to be called by his first name or nickname. This rule can be dropped when some familiarity is established and if the client addresses the worker by his/her first name. Undoubtedly, there are other valid exceptions to this rule, but these must be weighed within the context of the collaborative relationship between worker and client.

The range of counselling skills generally utilized by social workers are applicable to work with the frail elderly. Their cognitive deficits, not infrequently present, and general depletion, as characterized often by depression and anxiety, call for well-structured interviews, partializing of the problem; careful exploration of facts and feelings; clarification of what to the client may appear to be a jumble of ideas and feelings; and interpreting and summing up of what has transpired.

What may appear to be incoherent ramblings or reminiscences on the part of a frail client may indeed be part and parcel of a message he/she is trying to convey.[9] Active listening on the part of the worker is essential. Structure is introduced by the worker in such a way that the client does not feel ignored or thwarted in telling his/her story.

> Mr. L., 90-years-old, confused and depressed since his stroke, was wary about entering a nursing home but knew there was no other option for him. The social worker who visited him at the hospital wheeled his chair to a private office. She explained her purpose in seeing Mr. L.—to make plans for placement—but expressed her interest in how things were going for Mr. L. now. Mr. L. complained bitterly for over ½-hour about the way he was being treated in the hospital and his previous institutional experiences earlier in life, including the army and an orphanage. The worker later was able to refocus on the plan for placement having recognized with Mr. L. his fears of being in an authoritarian setting and suggesting they work together to look for a home where he would enjoy some independence.

Skilled interviewing enables the worker to establish a contract with the frail client, whose participation can vary depending on their degree of impairment. The contract can be simply to make an assessment or to work together on making friends in the nursing home. Clear, agreed-upon goals are as essential with the frail client as with younger healthier ones. Decline and very old age do not preempt the achievement of limited realistic goals.

Direct work on the part of the social worker with the frail client will continue until the goals of the contract are realized, i.e., setting up a plan of home care, placement in a nursing home, etc. The auxiliary function role demands, however, an extended commitment on the part of the social worker if there is no one else present to fill this role or if this significant other is incapacitated. As we have stressed, the vulnerability of the frail elder requires someone familiar, capable, and caring to be available in times of need.

Ongoing direct social work with the frail elder is particularly appropriate with the client who lacks in social skills or whose personality is such that others are repelled or rejected by him. The social worker's professionalism and understanding of the client's problems permit an ongoing alliance which others might not be able to tolerate.*

> Mr. P., 75-years-old, had been a lifelong alcoholic and now was seriously ill with cirrhosis and various other ailments. He was an angry, yet alternatingly ingratiating man who tended to "use" people as well as confuse them. He thus failed to form any lasting relationships. The worker who had achieved some trust because of her success in obtaining financial entitlements for him continued to keep contact with him on a monthly basis. Her familiarity with his communication problems helped her to serve as troubleshooter with neighbors and caretakers.

Interventions with Client Groups

Frailty and impairment do not diminish the need for social contacts, but they can interfere with the ability to form and sustain them. The risk of a frail elder being isolated from peers is great regardless of where he or she lives: alone, with family, or in a nursing home. The pattern of a client's previous social life as well as his or her own stated desires is a good indication of the need and type of socialization to be restored for the frail client.

The auxiliary function role may require direct work with the client to rekindle an interest in socialization particularly if the client has become withdrawn or fearful. It also requires very concrete steps to organize group activities which clients simply cannot physically do for themselves.

> The agency was providing home care services to a number of frail clients who benefited from this care but felt lonely and iso-

---

*For a detailed description of the techniques and skills in working with the frail elderly, the reader is referred to the authors' text, *The Auxiliary Function Model of Social Work Practice with the Frail Elderly and their Families.*

lated. A weekly meeting was organized at the agency for 8 clients. Their social workers encouraged participation. Transportation was organized for each as well as special provisions for personal care during the time away from home.

An important by-product of these group sessions is the ongoing relationships which are formed and sustained between meetings if only by telephone. Self-help in the form of reciprocally sharing the auxiliary function is even possible.

Problem-Solving with the Family

Very often the family is the client in our work with the frail elderly, both in the community and in the nursing home. In some instances the family—particularly the spouse or adult child—fills the auxiliary function role and is trusted by the frail elder to do so. In these cases most social work interventions are addressed to the family as a group.

In other instances the auxiliary role is shared with the family. Here a blend of individual and family group interventions is appropriate. In rare instances the family refuses to play the auxiliary role or the elder refuses to entrust this role to a family member. Special skills are called for which take into account the rights and integrity of all the adults involved.

When the auxiliary role is assumed by or shared with the family, a problem-solving strategy is called for which involves all significant family members, including the elder. The steps involved include: (1) convening family members (by phone if necessary); (2) giving every family member an opportunity to state his opinion and express his feelings about the situation; (3) seeking as much information as possible from the worker and outside resources; (4) with new information, re-examining and defining the problem or problems; (5) seeking commitments from family members on what they are able or not able realistically to do; (6) with all resources on hand, reaching a decision on a mutually agreed-upon plan; and (7) tapping the formal system, if necessary.

These steps in problem solving are not necessarily consecutive and may have to be repeated a number of times. What is most important is that they bring together on common ground the often disparate members of an elder's family who may have been haphazardly providing for care and help, to better organize their efforts.

Mrs. G. sought nursing home care for her mother—an 85-year-old, partially paralyzed stroke victim who had recently come to live with the G.'s after having lived with her oldest daughter for the past three years. Mrs. G. had impulsively offered to care for her mother out of anger toward her alcoholic husband, but now was terribly overburdened and only angrier at her husband. Other siblings and in-laws lived nearby and, although in years gone by had taken their turn in caring for the mother, were no longer eager to do so.

It quickly became apparent that for years old Mrs. G., since becoming widowed and ill, had been transferred from one child's home to another on an erratic basis depending on when the burden became too great or another problem in the family precipitated a change. There seemed little awareness on the part of any family members of the actual care needed by Mrs. G. and the nature of her difficulties. The agency who called home health aide services felt it would be best first to hold some family meetings which might achieve some coherent planning. After three family meetings it became clear that the widowed daughter could keep the mother in her home, which the mother wanted, with planned respite to be provided by other family members and home health aide service from the agency.

The decisions reached in family problem solving are not unilateral and, while never perfect solutions, can be owned by each member of the family, including the elder since they participated in the problem-solving process. A pattern is often set for future problem solving which invariably enriches the auxiliary function role of the family who can learn to move in and out of different problem situations as the needs of the elder dictate.

Service Systems and Community Interventions

Frailty and disability can affect the ability of elders not only to carry out tasks of daily living but to negotiate the various elements of the physical and social environment on which they have become more dependent. With family, friend, or neighbor the elder can be successful in establishing a helping network, although help is sometimes needed. As service systems become large and more bureaucratized, help more often than not is needed to negotiate them.

This help is an integral part of the auxiliary function comprising interpreting, advocacy, mediating, and coordinating transactions with service and community systems. The auxiliary function may be shared with others, i.e., the worker supplementing efforts of family or friend. It may involve transactions with the environment, in addition to family problem solving, to strengthen the relational aspects of the auxiliary function on the part of significant others.

Intervention with other service systems involves interdisciplinary collaboration. A wide range of other service providers, ranging from the physician to the chore worker, interact with the frail client. Understanding of the client's situation may vary widely since their view of his problem may come from a particular perspective, such as a medical one. The multifaceted nature of the client's problem—its biological, social, and psychological implications—may need to be stressed.

> The hospital team felt strongly that Mr. J. immediately needed a protective environment in view of his very poor health and mental confusion. The social worker was able to convey to the team the elderly patient's lifelong fear of dependency and the importance of allowing him to make the decision about his future life in his own manner and timing.

Less frail and depleted adult clients can more easily convey their needs to other disciplines. The sensory and mental impairments often suffered by the old, in addition to their general depletion, interfere with their ability to communicate. Perhaps most serious of all is the tendency of professionals and lay alike to discount the direct communications of the mentally impaired old person who is viewed as infantile, deranged, or simply incompetent. The interpretive and sometime mediating role of the worker provides an important link between client and the service system. It is also an enabling role in which the worker fosters better communications between the two. Both roles are critical aspects of the auxiliary function.

The bureaucratic and physical environments can effect this adaptation of the frail elderly, and interventions on the part of the social worker— often in the role of advocate—are required. Issues which must be addressed are manifold ranging from decent housing, transportation, income, and personal services to more subtle issues such as societal attitudes and organizational opportunities for socialization. These issues will be examined more closely as we examine the unique aspects of social work practice in home care and the nursing home.

Although, a case-by-case appraisal (including individual and environmental factors) is usually needed, interventions for the frail elderly are often better addressed on a group, community, organizational, and political level. These may be in tandem with or a substitution for individual efforts.

> Mrs. G., although receiving good care from the agency, was in a constant state of terror and anxiety over the lack of safety in her housing project. Other elderly clients were similarly affected, and the agency interceded with the housing management to provide better protection to the building. The worker also made special arrangements for an escort to accompany Mrs. G. on her visits to the clinic.

A caveat is in order at this junction and is applicable to all environmental transactions on behalf of the frail elderly. It relates to the fact that an overabundance of environmental inputs can be as harmful to the frail elderly as a scarcity of these inputs. The notion that "more is better" tends to pervade our work with the frail and may be a normal reaction to the depletion they exhibit. But, just as the worker (and family or friend) must exercise caution not to overprotect or infantilize in carrying out the auxiliary function, so must caution be exercised in transactions with the environment.

The client's own sense of control over the environment should not be diminished unless absolutely necessary or unless this is unimportant to him or her. Many transactions can be continued by the frail client with or without help from the worker.

> Mr. W., a cautious man and proudly independent, was obviously in need of meals and chore services. The worker helped him evolve a plan whereby he could purchase these services from local neighbors and thus feel he had some control over the situation. She took this approach although aware that the service might be less adequate than that which she could have arranged through the formal system.

Environmental inputs should not be excessive, robbing the client of the challenge required to exercise his remaining capacities. It is often

better to risk not stepping-in than have a task performed or service provided that the client can potentially do for himself or herself. "Excess
disability" on the part of the frail elderly has been cited as a common
problem referring to disabilities which cannot be accounted for by the
actual impairment of the elders but rather result from an overprotective
environment.[10]

The Home Care Setting

Care for the frail elder in his own home is characterized chiefly by
the fact that services are brought *to* the client, enabling him to retain
a real or perceived degree of independent living in the community. Even
if heavily dependent on the care of others, the community-based elder
usually experiences a greater sense of control over his life since he can
live with a modicum of flexibility and because of the symbolic meaning
of being on home ground. For some elders (and their frail spouses) this
sense of control is the chief motivation for remaining in the community
despite extreme disability. For others, the attachment to familiar surroundings and persons is a crucial factor.

The auxiliary function of the social worker in the home setting is
tempered by the balance which must be maintained between retaining the
positive features of community living, i.e., autonomy and/or familiarity, and the risks encountered by many frail elders. These risks are
related to unsafe neighborhoods, physical barriers, and the lack of 24-
hour supervision.

A strong collaborative relationship between worker and client can help
to maintain this balance. An ongoing process of problem solving can address crises before or as they arise. The active participation of the elder
in decision making and interaction with the worker help to mitigate any
sacrifices he might have to make.

> Mrs. P., 85-years-old, was holding on tenaciously to her home of
> 50 years and the privacy and familiarity it afforded her. She was
> eating poorly, however, and misusing her medications. The social
> worker's plan for regular visits from a nurse to supervise and
> monitor these activities were adamantly refused by Mrs. P. She
> trusted the worker enough, however, to talk about what she really
> feared: mainly, that an outsider would "take over." The worker
> in turn was able to assure Mrs. P. of the very limited tasks which
> the nurse would perform.

Home care, of course, encompasses services to the elder living with younger and/or healthier relatives who may provide auxiliary and care-taking functions. When these tasks are successfully carried out by family members or even friends and neighbors *respite care* may be all that is required to stabilize the situation.

Respite care may involve short-term placement of the elder in a nursing home or hospital to allow families a vacation. Day care is an excellent respite service. The utilization of home health aide services on an ad hoc or ongoing basis can give needed relief to caregivers.

Helping Networks

One of the chief differentiating features of the home care setting is that it is embedded in a larger community of greatly varying dimensions and resources which can be referred to as helping networks. When help-ing networks are not in place in the community—or if they are dis-organized or ineffective—it is incumbent on the social worker to mobilize and organize these resources if at all possible. Not only can some tasks be more efficiently performed by family, friend, or neighbor; but the ac-tive involvement of these informal supports is essential to a cost effective delivery of services to an ever growing frail population.

Situations can exist for community elders where family, friends, and neighbors are not fully aware of their plight. With the permission of the elder, the worker can serve as intermediary with these potential supports and through the problem-solving process organize care.

> Widowed Mrs. S., who had no children, was reluctant to burden a nearby niece with multiple needs arising from her increasing dis-ability. She permitted the worker, however, to contact her as well as some friendly neighbors. Neighbors were helped to organize a routine of shopping, meal preparation, and socialization. The niece, relieved that day-to-day care was provided, gave affective support through Sunday visits. The agency supplemented the care plan with a weekly homemaker.

In addition to providing care a member of the helping network may be able to assume the auxiliary function or share it with the worker. In the case of Mrs. S., she grew much closer to her niece and could con-fide in her. The niece, however, could not deal with the transactional aspects of the auxiliary function which the worker continued to perform.

The critical issue for the social worker in organizing helping networks in the community is the extent to which she or the agency remain involved. Three important criteria must be considered in making this decision. The first is the dependability of the helping network. If the helping network comprise other vulnerable elders, the worker might at the least continue to monitor the situation. Informal caretakers, although appearing to be interested, may be exploitive of the elder, and their help, if accepted at all, should be supervised.

Second is the nature of the tasks which have to be performed. Obviously, skilled nursing tasks cannot be performed by a neighbor. Homemaking and personal care particularly for a sick disabled person requires skill and supervision. Shopping, friendly visiting, and chores might be much more readily performed by an available neighbor.

Closely related is the third criterion—the behavior and personality of the elder. Skill is required in performing the auxiliary function for the elder who is mentally disturbed, depressed, or socially inept. The establishment of a collaborative relationship in and of itself is a challenge to professional skills. Since the environment may be hostile to this type of elder, the worker's transactional as well as relational skills may be required on an ongoing basis.

Each of these criteria must be considered in establishing a plan of home care in conjunction with the informal network and other agencies. If the plan of care provides for auxiliary and caretaking functions to be completely taken over by a community network, the worker can close the case. If doubt exists, the situation can be monitored on a regular basis.

In setting up a plan of homecare where formal caregivers remain involved, the social worker should transfer where possible the auxiliary function to the member of the helping team involved most with the client. This might include the nurse, a home health aide, or even volunteer friendly visitors. The latter, known as "community counselors" can carry out the function most effectively with support and help.[11]

Case Management

Case management is a term being increasingly used to describe services in home care akin to the social work function. Yet, there is little consensus on what case management really does include and whether or not it is a social work function. In fact, case managers are not always social workers.

In its simplest form case management refers to the organization, coordination, and monitoring of community services for a frail elder on the basis of a functional assessment. It does not necessarily include counselling as a discrete function. Case management gained its current popularity as a concept because of the fragmentation of community services and the need for a "manager" to expedite the delivery of services to the frail elderly.

From our perspective, case management is an important element of the auxiliary functional model. It refers to those instrumental tasks which the elder can no longer manage for himself temporarily or permanently and usually involving negotiations with the service system. It is *not* a model for social work practice with the frail elderly. It refers to a cluster of tasks which alone does not fully address their psychosocial problems.

By the same token case management tasks do not have to be carried out by the social worker. As we have noted, the auxiliary function can be a shared one. On the other hand, case management tasks may be the only ones being handled by the social worker.

> Mrs. J.'s 90-year-old mother had been living with her and her husband for 15 years. The couple were proud of the care and comfort they had been able to give the mother and the trust she placed in them. Both were now ailing and in need of some help but were thwarted at their attempts to get help. The only resource their family doctor could suggest was a nursing home. Confused and helpless about the service system, they turned to a worker at the local office on aging to help them negotiate the service systems and work out a more suitable home arrangement.

The other side of the "case management" coin is its administrative function. When a variety of services are organized for a frail elder, someone in the agency system must be "in charge" of a case. A variety of services may be provided by one agency, and if the service providers are organized into a team, the case manager becomes its captain. If services are provided by several different agencies, effective community collaboration dictates that someone be designated case manager to be accountable for a particular case insuring that the frail client does not "slip between the cracks."

Outreach

The auxiliary function model requires that attention be given to the frail elder who may be overlooked by the usual referral channels or is unable to seek help for himself. A system of outreach must be organized by agencies who serve the frail elderly to those persons or institutions in the community who might be aware of an elder in distress but unaware of how to help them.

These outreach targets might include physicians, housing managers, churches, hospital emergency rooms, postmen, and the elderly themselves. Outreach techniques might include local speaking engagements, door-to-door distributors of literature, and even TV and televised spots.

Identifying a frail elder in need does not necessarily mean they want help. If the situation is not a dangerous one, the most that can be done sometimes is to offer help and information. If the situation is dangerous, then extraordinary efforts on the part of the social worker may lead to some trust on the part of the frail elder and a willingness to accept help. Usually, in these situations the elder is depressed, suspicious, and irrational. Experienced protective service workers over the years have been effective in providing help which sidesteps the need for legal action.

> The superintendent was concerned about Mrs. F. who had become increasingly isolated, refusing to answer the door. Since she was so old and usually friendly, he decided to seek help. The worker attempted to seek access to Mrs. F.'s apartment, but was refused three times. She left brochures under the door and notes, to no avail. Since Easter was coming, she left a basket of Easter eggs and the next week was invited in. Eventually, Mrs. F. could accept services, and her condition and outlook improved immeasurably.

The Nursing Home

The most unique aspects of the nursing home in terms of social work practice are the totality, communality, and usually, the permanence of the setting. With great variations, these parameters of institutionalization are as true for the nursing home as the state hospital. Clients adapt to a social milieu which (with the exception of former state hospital patients) is very different from their life in the community.

Elderly clients are subject—24 hours a day—to the rules and regulations and role expectations which are required if care of a large number of patients is to be accomplished. They must share most aspects of their lives with other residents and, because of their age, infirmities, and lack of resources, find themselves permanently situated.

Nursing home placement is indeed a *social* experience for the frail elderly. Not only is it a very different social experience than their earlier lives, but the social aspects of nursing home care are, in many cases, the chief reason why nursing home placement has been sought: namely, the loss of supports in the community.

Although social work services in the nursing home are customarily considered secondary at best to nursing and medical care, their importance is paramount both in terms of helping clients adapt to a very different way of life, and for the frail in terms of ensuring the implementation of the auxiliary function. The protective environment of the nursing home may diminish the need for social work services or someone else who can fill the auxiliary function. In the case of a substandard nursing home, this need may be critical.

Even the most benign of nursing home environments, however, can fail to meet the need of the old person for a close relationship with another person. The depletion and depression which accompanies frailty and placement can impede the older person's aggressively forming such a relationship with staff or other residents. Direct intervention by the social worker and the formation of a strong working relationship temporarily or over a long period of time may be necessary, particularly if other ties cannot be formed.

> When Mr. L. was forced to enter a nursing home very much against his will, but out of necessity because of a disabling stroke, the worker quickly observed that his anger and mistrust would jeopardize his being accepted by staff and made concerted efforts to win his trust. He was able, after a period of time, to limit his angry outbursts to the times he was with the worker who, in turn, understood and accepted them. His behavior with other staff became less hostile, and his adjustment in the home seemed stabilized. Because of the precariousness of his feelings, the worker maintained close contact with him.

Family involvement does not cease with nursing home placement. Family members unable to care for the elder in the community will follow them into the nursing home and can be invaluable in filling an auxiliary function. Their involvement at times may be excessive or dysfunctional to the resident's adjustment and the skills of the social worker needed to channel their efforts constructively. The placement process itself can be a family problem-solving effort in which the social worker can play a helpful role.

Ongoing programs for families can be very helpful. The family's role in relation to an elder usually shifts when nursing home placement is made. Through group meetings or a family auxiliary, members of different families can help each other to make the transition.[12]

Group interventions for residents enhance individual functioning as well as provide a cost-effective method of service delivery in nursing homes. Natural groups are formed by those sharing living or dining space (and common problems arising from this) on a floor. Special interest groups in continuing education or living history can expand horizons. Because of varying areas of strength and weakness, residents can be helped to fill an auxiliary function for one another.

Even though surrounded by staff and other residents, the frail elder may lack the physical, mental, or emotional capacity to form relationships and socialize. Some staff—particularly those trained in therapeutic recreation—are sensitive to these problems and skillful in involving the frail person. But the social worker needs to be attentive to these needs as well as helping to maintaining distance for the resident who prefers and needs isolation.

Intake and Discharge

These are important social work functions, for they mark the transition from community into the nursing home and back into the community. Nursing home placement is often an irrevocable act for old persons since they usually give up their home in the community and have insufficient resources to return to the community if they choose to do so.

The decision to enter a nursing home, and to leave, therefore, is an extremely important one for a frail old person and, unfortunately, is made at a time when his or her decision-making capacities are at a low ebb. Mental impairment may interfere with the capacity to sort out facts and feelings and to study and weigh the pros and cons. Even if the frail clients' thinking capacities are completely intact, their physical and emotional condition may preclude effective decision making.

The client's participation in the intake and discharge processes is also an important precursor of his later adjustment. The need for an auxiliary other at this juncture is critical—a person who can closely align with the frail client's position. Family members are sometimes the least able to play this role, whether because their own needs are paramount or because they are overwhelmed by guilt. They need as much help as the elderly applicant, and family problem solving is very effective here.

Intake staff who are compelled to fill beds are also not appropriate for this role. The social worker, whether or not on the nursing home staff, is ideally suited, given a professional commitment to the needs of the client.

Short-term use of nursing homes may become increasingly popular if and when community services increase and improve for the frail elderly. Discharge planning must be initiated during the intake process and be an essential ingredient of care of the resident whose sights must be set on life back home and the changes ahead.

Organizational Change

Service systems and community interventions in the case of the nursing home very specifically apply to the administration and staff organization. The insular nature of nursing homes is both an advantage and drawback to social work efforts. On the positive side, organizational change can be clearly targeted. By the same token, intransience in the system affords the social worker few other options for achieving change.

Organizational change is sought in the nursing home for a variety of reasons: to change rules and regulations which are too restrictive; to enhance opportunities for staff enrichment and training; to increase communications among staff and between staff and patients. When the nursing home administrator is sensitive to social issues and to the special needs of the frail elderly, he or she usually welcomes social work input. If not, the social worker's task is a more involved one requiring a sensitivity to the needs and problems of administration and a clear grasp of how the administrator's needs and the social needs of the residents can coincide. For example, it can be pointed out that socially adjusted residents in nursing homes enhance the ambiance and attractiveness of a home; they are far easier to manage and thus, in the long run, less expensive to care for than agitated, depressed, and regressed residents who require a great deal of nursing and custodial care.

Another important target for organizational change in the nursing home is the floor team. The team formally or informally involves the nursing staff, physician, psychiatrist, physical and occupational therapists, the social worker, family members, and the elder. If organized to meet regularly for the purpose of coordinating resident care, these meetings can be an invaluable opportunity for social work input around a variety of issues as well as for gaining firsthand knowledge about residents' social problems. If not organized, the social worker should attempt to do so. While at first staff may be put off by what appears to be a time-consuming effort, they invariably come to value the usefulness of these meetings.

Resident Councils

Ways must be found in the nursing home environment wherein residents can regain or feel they have regained some control over their lives. The least restrictive the nursing home the better. A very minimum of rules and routine is necessary if client decision making is to be enhanced. Regardless of the degree of flexibility in rules and routine, the nursing home still looms large as an institutional force dominating the lives of residents, and organizational means should be provided which give them a sense of power in their everyday lives. A tried and tested method is the establishment of resident councils.[13]

The establishment of a resident council requires administrative fiat; otherwise it is powerless (unless an outside authority has sanctioned it). Specific meaningful tasks should be assigned to the council such as the design of activities, the approval of menus, etc. Opportunity should also be present for resident feedback, although care must be taken to avoid council meetings from becoming ineffective complaint sessions.

The social worker in her auxiliary role can help to organize a council, assisting with the practical details and holding regular elections. Councils can be simple or complex in structure and follow a variety of different types of structure. Most importantly they should be taken and treated seriously. Akin to the resident council is the family auxiliary which is organized in some homes (often by a social worker) to give families an opportunity for input into organizational matters.[14]

Priority Setting

While abuse or neglect of the elderly can occur in both the community and home care setting, current conditions in some nursing homes can be particularly challenging to the social worker who may be compelled to confront her own employer. We have noted the mediating and interpretive elements of the auxiliary function which can be carried out by the worker or resident council who seeks organizational change. When worker and residents, however, face an intransient situation, steps may have to be taken which can jeopardize the worker's employment. Legal consultation may be required as well as consultation with the National Association of Social Workers.

Short of situations of actual abuse or neglect, social workers face other problems. A particularly pressing one is shortage of staff. In some instances, the social worker may only serve as a consultant several hours a week. Social workers, if present at all, in nursing homes are pressed to prioritize their tasks and to weed out from their duties any activity which can be carried out by another person: resident, family, volunteers, or staff member.

This makes good sense not only because it is a cost-efficient use of the worker's time, but it fits comfortably into the auxiliary function model which seeks to strengthen or organize auxiliary aid for the frail elderly from as wide a network as possible. It is incumbent upon the worker to screen carefully the demands made upon her/him by staff, residents, or families. These demands may not coincide with actual needs.

> Mrs. F., a dependent, needy woman all her life, insisted that the worker visit with her often usually reporting one crisis after another. Actually, she was unusually able to fend for herself in the nursing home, and the worker withdrew her services.

By the same token, real need may exist where no demands are made.

> Mrs. S. had been confused and withdrawn since coming into the nursing home six months ago. An undemanding resident, the staff attributed her condition to senile dementia. Upon further exploration the worker discovered that Mrs. S. was acutely lonely but afraid to reach out because of her confusion. Gradually, with the worker's help, she was able to socialize more.

The worker may also choose to spend a significant amount of time in organizing helping networks in the home, social groups, and volunteer counsellors and concentrate on in-service staff training. Direct client interventions should be restricted to only the most complex, difficult situations which others cannot handle.

There is little question that the worker will have to make painful decisions about the allocation of time, neglecting some residents who truly need professional help. These unmet needs should be carefully documented and brought to the attention of the administrator and/or others potentially able to increase staff.

Summary

Our basic premise is that the problems of the frail elderly client, which are closely related to depletion and loss, determine the social work function both in the nursing home and home care setting. This social work function has been described as an auxiliary one: providing a helping relationship and transactional links with the environment on a continuing or as-needed basis. These affective and instrumental elements of the auxiliary function are shared with other formal and informal supports, a complementarity determined by the capacities of the elder, the resources of the environment, and the tasks to be performed. The social worker's unique tasks are to identify, organize, and support these significant others and to assume the auxiliary function in lieu of available others. The "study, assessment, and plan"; direct practice skills with client and client groups; problem solving with the family; and service systems and community interventions are relevant to practice regardless of the setting.

Striking organizational differences in the nursing home and home care settings, inherent in their organizational structures of by-products of current conditions require special interventions. The home care setting is embedded in a larger community of widely varying dimensions. While it affords the frail elderly a greater degree of real or perceived freedom and continuity of life-style, it requires case management skills to orchestrate a variety of informal and formal resources and establish a helping network. The implementation of the auxiliary function in the form of outreach is particularly critical in the case of the isolated frail elder.

The nursing home setting is a far less open system offering the advantages of 24-hour protection and a contained service community which hypothetically reduces the need for implementing the auxiliary function. Certain inherent organizational features, however, are antithetical to the differing needs of the clients for autonomy, emotional intimacy, and individualization, requiring that the auxiliary function be implemented on an individual level with attention to intake and discharge and on the group and organizational level through resident groups and councils and floor teams. Poor conditions in a number of nursing homes on which elders are totally dependent call for priority setting and special advocacy and mediating skills on the part of the social worker.

Regardless of the setting in which the auxiliary function model is practiced, it is undergirded by the principles and ethics of the social work profession. Client self-determination and actualization are no less compelling with the frail, depleted elder than with younger and healthier persons whose biological potential for growth and change is greater. The challenge to the social worker is to pursue relentlessly that crucial balance between autonomy and dependency which benefits the frail elder.[15]

REFERENCES

1. Brody, Elaine M. *Long-Term Care of Older People: A Practical Guide.* New York: Human Sciences Press, 1977, pp. 28-40.

2. Brody, Elaine M. "Long-Term Care of the Aged: Promises and Prospects. *Health and Social Work*, February 1979, pp. 29-59.

3. Long-Term Care Task Force, NCSW. *The Future of Long-Term Care in the United States.* Washington, D.C.: U.S. Department of Health, Education and Welfare, February 1977.

4. Miller, D. B. "The Role of the Social Worker in Long-Term Care." *Journal of the American Health Care Association, 21* (7), 1980, pp. 95-100.

5. Long-Term Care Task Force, NCSW. *The Future of Long-Term Care in the United States.* Washington, D.C.: U.S. Department of Health, Education and Welfare, February 1977.

6. Goldfarb, Alvin I. "Patient-Doctor Relationship in Treatment of Aged Persons." *Geriatrics*, January 1964.

7. Germaine, Carol B. and Gitterman, Alex. *The Life Model of Social Work Practice.* New York: Columbia University Press, 1980.

8. Wasser, Edna, *Creative Approaches in Casework with the Elderly.* New York: Family Services Association of America, 1975.

9. Liton, Judith and Olstein, Sara C. "Therapeutic Aspects of Reminiscence." *Social Casework, 50* (5), 1969, pp. 263-268.

10. Brody, E. M., Cole, C., and Moss, M. "Individualizing Therapy for the Mentally Impaired Aged." *Social Casework, 54* (8), 1973, pp. 453-461.

11. Greengross, Sally. "Aging and the Community Counsellor." In *Impact of Aging: Strategies for Care*, David Holman, Ed. New York: St. Martin's Press, 1981, p. 128.

12. Silverstone, Barbara M. "The Family Is Here to Stay." *Journal of Nursing Administration*, May 1978.

13. Silverstone, Barbara M. *Establishing Resident Councils.* New York: Federation of Protestant Welfare Agencies, 1972.

14. Silverstone, Barbara M. "The Family Is Here to Stay." *Journal of Nursing Administration*, May 1978.

15. Stevenson, Olive. "Caring and Dependency." In *Impact of Aging: Strategies for Care*, David Holman, Ed. New York: St. Martin's Press, 1981, pp. 158-175.

Chapter 2

THE HOSPITAL CENTER AND AGING: A CHALLENGE FOR THE SOCIAL WORKER

Susan Blumenfield

Despite what may seem like a paradox, no volume on gerontological social work in long-term care would be complete without a discussion of practice in the acute care hospital. By definition, hospitalization in the acute setting is not long term. However, it is necessary to conceptualize the acute hospital as part of any system of long-term care for older people.

However short in time, a hospitalization may be pivotal in the life of any individual. Illness or accident may lead to a change in functioning of the older person, a breakdown in supports the person has had, a change in the social support system he or she needs, a need for a changed living situation, or alterations in the feelings of vulnerability and self-esteem. The hospital is often the setting for fear, pain, even death. It may be the ray of hope for cure or palliation of discomfort. Whatever occurs, the hospital is not an insignificant experience for the people who are treated there and clearly plays a role in the long-term care of older people.

It is almost inevitable that older people will have to spend some time in the hospital. "Older people have high rates of illness and disability and a high demand for health services."[1] They make up a large proportion of people cared for in hospitals and need longer and costlier care than the under-65-year-old population. In 1973, the average length of hospital stay for those 65 and over was 12.1 days. For those 15-44, it was 5.7 days.[2] People 65 and over make up 11% of the population but accounted for 29% of the bill for personal health care.[3] Hospital care is a costly but ever present reality, particularly in late life.

Because chances of hospitalization at some point in late life are so high, the hospital may actually be the point of entry in the health care system for many older people. It is during an acute hospitalization that many older people not only develop specific needs for services, but many have had needs which only during a hospital stay are recognized and addressed. Hospital social workers provide the linkages necessary to obtain services both from within the institution and from outside the specific hospital. The fact that the hospital is often a point of access to other services makes it an important component of long-term care of the elderly and a major setting for gerontological social work practice.

A final rationale for the discussion of practice in the acute hospital in this volume is the fact that the hospital setting is a microcosm of society. Attitudes that people hold toward the elderly carry over into this setting. While the hospital is a discrete institution providing total care for a period of time, it also remains a part of the community where care of any patient is influenced by many outside forces. Of necessity social work practice with older people in this setting takes on a long-term care perspective.

Social work in the acute care hospital has a primary care focus. It is the social work discipline that takes on the coordinating function with the goal of preventing breakdown due to remediable social causes. Social work is also practiced with a population receiving outpatient medical care. Such work is part of the long-term care of older people. While there is not space in this chapter to go into this arena in detail, it is important to note that it is a major focus for primary care and that many of the principles and issues discussed here are applicable also to outpatient work.

The Nature of the Hospital Setting

Before we look further at the social work function, we must look more closely at the acute hospital itself. John Knowles, in writing about the climate of the hospital, has stated:

> Progress in medical science and in the specialized division of medical skills has changed medicine from an individual intuitive enterprise into a social service. The hospital is the institutional form of this special service. It has developed from a house of despair for the sick poor to a house of hope for all social and economic classes in just the past 60 years.[4]

The general hospital today is a highly technical, high cost, acute care institution. The subdivision of labor has increased with the rise in technological advances. This has contributed to a "fragmented machine approach to the patient and dehumanizes what should be an intensely personal and humane encounter."[5] The evolution of the hospital from a palliative house for the poor and weary, to a high-powered curative center for the ill has undoubtedly been advantageous for mankind. "It is the spin-offs from this evolution that stimulates some wish for just a piece of the palliative qualities that once existed, particularly in the care of the old and chronically ill."[6]

Medical sociologists have explored the patient perceptions of their place in the hospital structure.[7] They have verified the feelings of dependency engendered by hospital routines and the feeling of vulnerability experienced by people awaiting procedures or medications. The waiting and the shedding of possessions, clothing, and control upon admission begins the process of depersonalization and dependency. Staying in the hospital fosters dependency and generally leads the patient to try to maintain him/herself in good standing with those in charge.[8] The patient soon learns what behaviors are rewarded and often feels as though he or she must comply in order to get the care he or she needs.

The older person entering the acute hospital quickly becomes enmeshed in this culture and may even suffer more because he or she is old. Stereotypical responses to older people may exacerbate the indignities. Such patients are often perceived by staff as an unrewarding drain on their limited resources. Frequently, the older person is robbed of his/her decision-making role. Personnel may treat the older person as if he or she is too old to understand, to contribute to planning for his/her care, or unable to respond to his/her surroundings. The fact that confusion can be a temporary result of illness is often not acknowledged. Younger patients seem to engender more frequent and more interested contacts with health care personnel than older patients. Thus, the older person occupies a position of even greater disadvantages than a younger person within the acute care setting.

Impact of the Hospital Setting on Social Work Practice

In the hospital, social work is one of many disciplines which are involved in caring for the patient. The fact that social work is practiced within a "host" institution effects how and what it can accomplish. The social worker will not be the only professional speaking with the patient, gathering information about the patient's functioning, and psychosocial concerns, but how the information is gathered, the assessment that is made, and the intervention of the social worker will be unique. Each discipline has its particular contribution to make toward the diagnosis and treatment of the patient. Social work practice in the hospital must be accomplished in collaboration with other hospital personnel.

While the biopsychosocial model of patient care is always relevant,[9] the hospital setting makes the recognition of this particularly important. The nature of the person's physical condition and its impact on his or her functioning must always be taken into account.

The hospital setting leads to the possibility of disequilibrium for older people in particular areas of which the social worker must be cognizant. Research has been done on the types of problems which social workers frequently work on with older hospital patients.[10] Such problems generally include those regarding adjustment to the hospital environment or change in functioning, as well as issues involved in planning for discharge and/or transitions in role relationships.

Social work practice with older people in the hospital not only involves the particular patient but includes the patient's family or significant others. The hospital social worker works with hospital personnel in a variety of ways but also works with personnel from community agencies, long-term care institutions, policy-making bodies, and advocacy groups. The social worker in the hospital must often coordinate services both within and outside the institution and must help to balance the needs of the numerous people involved with the patient.

To add to all of the foregoing areas in which the acute setting will have an impact on social work practice is the pervasive one that the work will generally occur in conditions of crisis and severe time limits. Short-term crisis intervention becomes the often used treatment modality. This is not only because illness is a crisis, but also because of the short lengths of stay and acute nature of the problems. Much needs to be accomplished in a short time.

The Older Hospitalized Patient as Part of a Special Population Group

Aging is part of the life cycle. It is a stage of growth, as Erikson tells us, with its own developmental tasks of maintaining a "sense of integrity" rather than a "sense of despair."[11] Hospitalization has a major impact during this life stage. How it will affect any individual is of course idiosyncratic and personal depending upon health status, income, family circumstances, culture, and personality.

Yet, we can separate the aged as a special population group to be considered because of special common concerns and needs which have a particular impact on the health care system. Of major import is the increasing number of people 65 years and over, and even more significant is the increasing percentage of this group who are over 75 years.

Another reason to consider the aged as a special population group is the extent of disability this group suffers. While most old people function quite well, the elderly, as a group, constitute the most disabled and impaired segment of the total population. Compared to younger groups, the ailments of older people are less often acute and more often characterized by multidiseases, chronic ailments, and disabling conditions. About 80% of those 65 and over have at least one chronic condition, about half, two or more.[12] Chronic illness is often accompanied by some impairment in function, and increasing age generally leads to greater impairment. Sensory deficits which rise with age can further complicate the effects of illness. These characteristics contribute to producing incongruence between older patients and the acute hospital which is organized to provide diagnosis and cure as rapidly as possible.

The aged can be identified as a special group not only because of numbers, chronicity of medical problems, and disability, but also, because there are age-related changes which cause some diseases to present in ways atypical for younger populations, many drugs to be metabolized differently and an even greater interaction of physical and mental illnesses than occur with younger people.[13] The aged also suffer disproportionately with problems of confusion, incontinence, and immobility as accompaniments to illness. Etiologies of these disorders are frequently difficult to find and difficult to treat. All of these issues have a strong impact on how the older person will interface with the acute hospital system.

Attitudinal issues often set the elderly apart as a special group. As has been discussed, older people, more than those at any other life stage, have been viewed as a homogeneous group. Stereotypical notions often color the perceptions of health personnel and can determine how they intervene.[14] This element is an overriding concern when looking at gerontological social work practice in the acute hospital setting.

Impact of Gerontological Social Work
in the Hospital on the Social Worker

Any setting and population group have an effect on the people providing service. Working with older people in the hospital has some striking dimensions which need to be explicated.

The social worker is confronted by older people who are often at major crisis points in their lives. For many, the hospital stay may mark a change in their functioning, even in their independence. It is an emotionally difficult task to help people at such transitions.

Gerontological social work in the hospital is, by definition, complex. There is much history, often a scattered, not easily identifiable support system, and a great number of variables to explore in the assessment process. Work with family members or supportive others is the rule, not an occasional change in role. Collaboration with other disciplines is a necessity.

The interplay of physical and emotional problems is striking in the older hospital patient, and the social worker is witness to the impact of social problems on the disease process and outcome for the older person. Working with a patient who dies is not an infrequent experience.

Social workers in the hospital are also not exempt from the therapeutic nihilism which can afflict other health care professionals with regard to the elderly.[15] They, too, may feel that time spent on the elderly is un-rewarding or unwarranted because of the likelihood that the older person has little time left.[16] They, too, may feel that working with the elderly has less status than working with other age groups who have greater status in society. They, too, may have accepted the myths of aging that would have them believe that the elderly routinely suffer from psycho-logical decline, social ineptitude, physical decay, and family abandon-ment. However, in the acute hospital setting, even though the social worker may not have chosen to work with the elderly, he or she cannot avoid the older patient. The patient will frequently have many needs for social service. Gerontological social work in the acute hospital setting therefore is practiced often with conflicted feelings about older people and a lack of previous interest in the area.

Hospital social workers are often much younger than the hospitalized elderly patient. They may have had much narrower real life experience with this age group than with any other. Thus, they may be influenced more by their own limited experience with grandparents or transferential feelings which arise in relation to this population.

In addition conflict is inherent in gerontological social work in the acute setting because of the complexity and time-consuming nature of such work in an environment that has heavy workloads, conflicting de-mands and limitations in time. One seldom works exclusively with older patients in the acute setting. Thus, balancing the needs of a variety of populations adds to the difficulties of providing optimal service for this particular group.

Always being confronted with illness and disability produces feelings of vulnerability in the worker. Frustration can be particularly high when dealing with a population where not all problems can be resolved or even alleviated. The realities of chronic illness, of fragmented and inadequate services for meeting needs, and of societal deficits have a major impact on work with older people in the acute setting. All of these make up the dilemmas and challenges of gerontological social work in the hospital.

Practice in the Acute Care Hospital

Gerontological social work in the hospital setting involves four major components:

1. Aiding adjustment of patient/family to hospitalization and illness.
2. Providing assistance in discharge planning.
3. Educating other staff about needs of older patients as well as of the particular patient.
4. Providing support for other staff involved in caring for older patients.

Each of these elements involves particular knowledge of the setting and the specific population as well as the utilization of generic social work skills in assessment and intervention.

Assessment

Assessment information is that which helps us look at the impact of an illness on a patient/family, in order to provide service where it is needed. In any assessment, we are dealing with the characteristics of the person/family, the illness, the environment, the social system, the needs of the person/family, and the resources available. It is the interaction of these characteristics which will contribute to the ability of the patient to function.

The assessment will be derived from how the following questions can be answered.

1. What is the illness?
2. Who is the patient? Family?
3. What are the strengths of the patient/family?
4. What are the needs of the patient/family?
5. What kinds of problems does patient/family have?

6. What kinds of help does the patient/family need?
7. Who in the environment can provide help?
8. What formal services can be brought to bear on patient/family needs?

Answers to these questions will always have a dynamic quality, as hospitalization is a crisis situation. Assessment needs to consider the past, the present, and the prognosis for the future. The social worker cannot hope to have total information about any patient at any particular time, but listed in Tables I, II and III are suggestions for areas in which information is most relevant in making an assessment of the patient and family.

Interventions in regard to aiding the patient's adjustment and discharge planning, as well as where education and/or support of other staff is needed, can be planned from the results of the assessment.

TABLE I

Patient Characteristics

1. Demographic Data

   Age
   Sex
   Race
   Religion
   Socioeconomic status
   Place of birth
   Language most comfortable in
   How supported financially
   Receiving or eligible for entitlements

2. Illness Data

   Diagnosis
   Prognosis
   Life-threatening?
   Change in Functioning?

3. Functional Data

   Ability in ADL
   Mental Status

Previous Functioning
ADL
Home Management
Social Interactions
Financial Management

4. Living Arrangements

Where living
With whom
Type of environment
Who available there to help
Safety
Accessibility

5. Social World

Who makes up social world of patient
Number of friends
How often seen
How helpful
Activities shared
Groups to which patient belongs

6. History

Education
Work history
Marital (family) history
Relationships with other
Areas in which patient had interests and found pleasure

7. Personality Characteristics

Coping style
Motivation
Flexibility
Expectations of self
                others
                system
Ability to use services

TABLE II

Informal Support System Characteristics

1. Family

   Who is in Family?
   >   relationship
   >   age
   >   particular situation

   Where do family members live?
   Who is available to the patient and for what?
   How willing is family to give support to patient?
   What are difficulties family has in helping patient?
   Is family able to help patient?
   What would help family in giving support to patient?
   What is assessment of family interaction?
   Family history with patient.
   What would be appropriate roles for family members in helping patient?

2. Neighbors/Friends

   Who does patient count on for help in the neighborhood?
   What are capacities and limitations of these neighbors/friends for helping?
   What kinds of services do neighbors/friends provide?
   How can they be supported in giving help?

3. Informal Groups—How can they be of help?

   Church groups
   Volunteers

TABLE III

Formal System

1. Eligibility for Entitlements?

   Medicare
   Medicaid
   S.S.I.
   Social Security

2. What services might be needed for patient out-of hospital

How to apply
Time lapse
Eligibility
Family involvement
How to facilitate application procedures

Intervention Strategies

1. Adjustment to Hospitalization and Illness

The Patient. When the social work assessment determines that the older person has particular problems adjusting to the hospital or illness, we need to work with the patient, family and the environment. The social worker provides a consistent and understanding relationship. The worker helps to individualize this patient through assessment and the interpretation to other staff of this particular patient's needs. The social worker increases the patient's understanding of the hospital environment and facilitates ways to meet the patient's idiosyncratic needs within the institution. Often social workers must slow the rapid-fire pace of activities in the hospital, for the patient, by interceding to be sure procedures and regimen are explained by the physicians and understood by the patient. We work to understand who the patient is and how he/she is reacting to the crisis of this hospitalization. The following example will illustrate some of these elements.

> Ms. P. was a 77-year-old, white single woman who was admitted to the hospital with cancer of a kidney, intractable back pain, and immobility. She was seen by medical staff as an angry, difficult woman and was referred to the social worker because she was refusing diagnostic tests and was difficult to deal with.
>
> When the social worker came to introduce herself to Ms. P. it was striking how the emaciated, pale Ms. P. almost blended in with the bedsheets that she was bundled up under. It was her clear mind, decisive speech, and angry flavor which made her noticeable. Ms. P.'s initial response to the social worker was that she needed no help from anyone who could not relieve her pain. The social worker acknowledged Ms. P.'s disappointment at not feeling helped, but persisted in her interest in Ms. P. It became evident

that Ms. P. felt thwarted and out of control because of her illness and helplessness in the hospital. To return some measure of control to Ms. P., the social worker suggested making an appointment to return for a longer conversation at a time to be chosen by Ms. P. The patient reluctantly agreed, but still appeared angry and disinterested. When the social worker offered her hand in parting, Ms. P. took it and allowed a faint smile to mark the beginning of an important relationship.

The social worker met with Ms. P. consistently for short periods almost everyday, during the patient's hospitalization. She was able to help Ms. P. regain some control in ways other then denying permission for diagnostic tests. This was accomplished by interpreting this need to staff who were able to create other areas of choice for Ms. P. They allowed Ms. P. to choose when she would sit up, when to have inbetween snacks, etc.

Ms. P. was understood as a woman who had been functioning independently all her life. She had worked as a bookkeeper until her retirement about 10 years earlier, and had lived with her sister in an apartment all her adult life. About 2 years prior to this hospital admission, Ms. P.'s sister had become ill with cancer. Ms. P. cared for this sister until the sister's death 4 months previously and had, herself, gone into a severe decline since then. Ms. P. expressed the theory that working so hard caring for her sister was actually the cause of her own present illness. Ms. P. needed to deal with the anger toward this deceased sister and that she, herself, was now ill with no one left to care for her.

Ms. P.'s fear of the dependency she felt led her to defend against such feelings by pushing people away who were trying to help. Ms. P. was helped by the social worker to understand some of these feelings. Simultaneously, the social worker met with staff to share her assessment of Ms. P.'s coping style and needs. This helped those working with Ms. P. to understand her anger and not to feel personally attacked. Tension lessened within the environment for Ms. P. at the same time that she was using the casework relationship for support and understanding.

Adjustment to the hospital often depends on helping the patient with concerns about things outside of the hospital. The older person, admitted to the hospital on an emergency basis, for example, might be demanding to return home prematurely in order to get a check or pay the rent.

If there is no immediately accessible "responsible other," the social worker must often take on this role or coordinate the services of others, which can contribute to the patient's peace of mind while in the hospital.

The Family. Often the social worker must work even more closely with a family member. While the older patient is ill and receiving treatment, it is sometimes a family member who has difficulty accepting the illness, the hospitalization or the treatment. The family member, by overt actions or covert sabotage, may interfere with the patient's care. The social work role is to understand the meaning of such behavior and work with family members and staff to resolve these problems.

Mrs. M. was an 87-year-old, Orthodox Jewish widow, admitted to the hospital for internal bleeding and anemia. Mrs. M. had been living at home, suffering from a variety of chronic conditions. She had been cared for by an 8 hour/day home attendant. Overseeing her care was her 57-year-old, married son, who lived nearby.

During the patient's hospitalization, her son stayed at the hospital all day, everyday. Mrs. M. suffered one medical crisis after another with the physician needing to do a variety of procedures and nursing staff being particularly attentive. The patient was quite ill and inaccessible to interview. Mr. M. spent most of the time reading religious books, but would jump up to meet any physician or nurse entering his mother's room to ask questions, suggest changes in procedures or discuss the merits of particular foods for his mother. Staff began to avoid entering Mrs. M.'s room, unless absolutely necessary. They also had problems restraining Mr. M. from feeding his mother. Staff had warned Mr. M. of risks in trying to give his mother food since she was restricted to a special diet. However, he persisted in trying to urge her to eat ice cream or soup brought from outside. Staff became frustrated and angry in trying to deal with the son both because of his behavior in the hospital and their belief that he was acting out of guilt for having let his mother become so ill before being brought to the hospital.

The unit social worker was asked to see Mr. M. to help staff deal with the problems. Mr. M. was difficult to get to know. His orthodoxy contributed to the discomfort he had speaking with women and the social worker needed to respect such feelings. He was eventually able to respond to discussion about his concerns and needs and explained how fearful he was of the discomfort his mother was having, and his anger that the doctors couldn't seem to do more for her. He felt that no one was talking to him and that he was helpless in the situation, for he never knew when the physician would be around or when something new would happen. Mr. M. was almost frantic in his need to do something. Praying in the hall outside his mother's room was one thing he felt he could do, as was trying to force her to eat in order to regain strength.

The social worker met with staff and was able to reframe Mr. M.'s behavior to the staff, from that of inscrutable, angry and ungrateful, to frightened, overwhelmed, and lacking direction. House staff and nurses were engaged in considering ways to help Mr. M. with his problems while attempting to do the most they could for the patient. It was agreed that the intern in charge of Mrs. M.'s care would schedule a specific time each day to meet with Mr. M. Setting limits on Mr. M.'s demands, yet attempting to give him information and support appropriately was suggested by the social worker as a way of providing structure that would help the patient's son.

The social worker also suggested that they attempt to find some roles for Mr. M. to fill his need to do something. It was suggested that Mr. M. read to his mother and help feed her the specific diet provided by the hospital.

By providing more understanding of the patient's son and how meeting his needs could help in caring for the patient, the social worker was able to engage the staff in thinking creatively together. Providing structure in which to work with this family member and some role for him to play helped him to cope with the hospitalization of his mother and be ready to actively help in planning for his mother's eventual discharge.

The acute care hospital often seems a forbidding place to the outsider. Activity appears fast-paced and intense, and patients and families are often intimidated and overwhelmed. The social worker needs to be aware of such feelings on the part of patients and families and be able to bridge the gap between outside world and the high-powered institution. The social worker must often help patients to communicate with other health care personnel. Unscrambling medical jargon can be a difficult task. The social worker can assist the patient and family by helping them to ask questions of the physician or to make lists of concerns so these can be addressed.

Seemingly simple tasks of orienting patients and families to routines and procedures, helping to direct them to facilities and personnel who could be of assistance within the hospital are often overlooked. The social worker must remain aware of how important these are in the hospital adjustment process.

The social worker in the acute care hospital often provides the linkage for the older patient and family with both the institution and the outside. There is always the need to balance the needs of patient and family with their own capacities and the resources available to them in the environment.

2. Discharge Planning

Discharge planning is a major role of the hospital social worker, particularly when working with older people. The hospital, though a temporary experience, is one with major consequences for future functioning.

In order to help patients in planning for discharge, the social worker must be aware of the previous functioning of the patient. The worker must understand the patient's physical condition and any changes in functioning that will occur because of it. Collaboration with medicine, nursing, physical therapy, etc., is essential in assessing the patient's medical condition, prognosis, ability to handle activities of daily living and to sustain care. It is important to share with other staff the social work assessment of the patient's mental status, emotional state, informal supports, and possible formal supports. It is the combined assessment by all the various professionals involved, together with the capacities and wishes of the patient and family, which lead, ultimately, to the plan for care following hospitalization.

When the social worker is involved with the hospital patient, he or she must balance conflicting demands and pressures around planning for discharge. The case of Mr. G. is an example of finding such a balance.

> Mr. G. came to the hospital quite confused, weak, and unable to walk. He was a 72-year-old, Hispanic man whose wife had died 8 years before and who had been living since that time with one of his married daughters. Upon his admission to the hospital, the daughter spoke to the social worker and discussed her feelings of being overwhelmed with his care and her inability to go on providing such care. Her own children aged 4, 8, and 10 needed her attention, the space in her apartment was cramped and tensions had increased between her and her husband.

Throughout Mr. G.'s hospitalization, his daughter's plaintive cry ran in counterpoint to his continuing improvement. Mr. G. proved a rewarding patient for staff. With medication changes, and improvement in the heart problems, Mr. G.'s mental status improved. He remained with moderate disorientation and confusion, but was able to respond appropriately in general and evidenced an engaging personality. He was cheerful, optimistic and amusing. With a great deal of nursing input, Mr. G. started to walk and provide his self-care with minimal assistance.

With the dramatic improvement, everyone was hopeful that Mr. G. could return to live with his daughter. All staff, including the unit social worker, began to press for such a discharge plan. However, the daughter, while guilty and most unhappy, remained adamont that Mr. G. could not continue to live in her apartment. The social worker began to receive calls from another daughter and son of the patient and was able to arrange a meeting with all the patient's children who were clearly at odds around the planning.

Mr. G. expected to return to his daughter's, although he acknowledged that his grandchildren were sometimes loud and bothersome. He also thrived on the attention given him by staff and responded to the interchange with the other patients in his room.

The social worker needed to help the family sort out their conflicting needs in regard to the patient. All three adult children were unhappy about sending their father to a nursing home, yet the brother and single sister could not agree to provide either a home or more aid for their father. The daughter who had been caring for him was still viewed as the logical person to continue such care, but her plight became clearer as they met together. Finding Mr. G. an apartment of his own and providing help there was ruled out as something not only difficult to do but something he had been unable to adjust to even years earlier. The fact that now, although appealing, Mr. G. needed direction, assistance, and help in orientation 24 hours-a-day made such a plan quite unrealistic.

The family agreed to apply for admission to an HRF near them so they could visit frequently. They found it difficult to discuss these plans with Mr. G. and needed help in including him in the planning.

The social worker was pressured by the family to "go ahead and make the arrangements." She was also pressured by the staff who were invested in this patient and who felt nursing home placement was inappropriate. The patient, himself, while speaking of returning to his daughter's was also somewhat aware of his comfort in the hospital. The social worker, herself, was not without bias and wanted this patient, who had improved so much, to return to the community.

However, the role of the social worker in planning discharge is to help to effect what is possible once the needs of the patient and resources at his disposal are known. The social worker had to work with the family to help them come to a plan of action. At the same time she helped them discuss this plan directly with the patient. Mr. G. was initially unhappy with the thought of not returning to his daughter's home. Because of the chance she had had to work through some of her ambivalent feelings with the social worker, the daughter was able to cope with Mr. G.'s disappointment and to help him see some positives in the proposal. The possibility of this being a temporary plan was also discussed.

The social worker also had to work with staff who were angry at this plan, and therefore at her for "allowing" it. The fact that families cannot be "told" what to do, as well as the ramifications of this particular family's interactions, were shared with staff. The feelings of investment in this patient and the fears that his improvement was "wasted" had to be acknowledged and dealt with. The social worker had to help staff see that the ways in which the hospital experience had been so positive for Mr. G. were features that would continue in a long term institution.

Another major area of work with older patients in the hospital is helping them to obtain entitlements. The social worker must be familiar with programs of benefits for older people and ready to assist them. A person often enters the health care system through the hospital. Thus it is in this institution, that he or she may be linked to other services which can be helpful.

In discharge planning, a person's eligibility for governmental programs like Medicaid, S.S.I., rent subsidies, etc., need to be assessed. Depending upon the financial situation as well as health care need, services may or may not be available to the particular patient. Often the social worker must act as an advocate to help the patient obtain needed services. The following case will illustrate such a situation.

Mrs. F., 73-year-old black widow, living alone, came to the hospital for rectal surgery. Mrs. F. had been managing alone with the help of a woman, sent by a local Title III agency, who helped with housework 4 hours a week. Mrs. F. while independent, had become increasingly limited in mobility due to arthritis, a hip problem, diabetes, and now bowel problems. Neighbors were helpful as was her married daughter. The latter, however, lived 3/4-hour away and had family responsibilities which included a 12-year-old, handicapped child.

Even before the surgery, Mrs. F. clearly needed more help at home and she had been assisted by the social worker in applying for Medicaid and for home help. These applications were already completed and approval verbally given prior to her short hospitalization. Both patient and daughter had been involved in this planning. There had been set backs and difficulties which the hospital social worker had helped them through and all seemed to be in place when Mrs. F. was discharged from the hospital. Mrs. F. was planning to spend a few days recuperating at her daughter's apartment before returning to her own apartment.

The day after discharge the social worker received a frantic phone call from the patient's daughter informing her that the Visiting Nurse Service that came would be unable to provide the health aide as expected because this could not be covered under Medicare. They needed the last three digits of the Medicaid number or could not process the billing. What followed this phone call was the bureaucratic nightmare that can discourage even the strongest of families and is all too often part of working with older people in the hospital.

The social worker had to verify the fact that the service was being withheld and attempted to advocate for the patient. She tried to get the necessary information from the Department of Social Services, but was unsuccessful. It seemed that there was no way to revive the original plan.

In order to provide Mrs. F. with interim help so that she could return home, a dozen agencies were contacted by the social worker and possibilities discussed for how a package of services could be created for Mrs. F. while she awaited receipt of her Medicaid card and placement of a DSS Home Attendant. Eventually, by combining limited services from a few separate agencies, on this short-term basis, Mrs. F. was able to return home. Through the major efforts of the hospital social worker, Mrs. F. regained her independence and her daughter respite which allowed her to continue to be available to provide support when needed.

This case illustrates one of the time-consuming, yet very important roles of the social worker regarding older people in hospitals; that of coordinating services and advocating for creativity in meeting a patient's needs.

The social worker in the hospital setting must be familiar with resources in the community and skilled at interpreting the needs of patients to outside agency personnel. Even with this knowledge and skill, all situations cannot be resolved as the one illustrated here. Often because of the various funding sources, vagaries of eligibility requirements or prohibitive costs, patients do not have access to services that they need. Working within this complex system is both challenging and frustrating.

Helping the patient/family become aware of and use resources that are available demands a special blend of knowledge and skill. Working on meeting a concrete need is often an important entre to the patient. Engaging on work together to obtain resources, the social worker can develop a relationship with the patient. The patient can experience the assistance of the social worker as helpful at the same time as it supports his or her autonomy and self-esteem. Such experience can lay the foundation for further work together in other areas of need.

The social worker in the acute hospital may have to deal with patients who evidence major symptoms of confusion and/or disorientation. Part of the social work role, initially, is to advocate for the examination of reversible causes of these symptoms. In those situations where it is determined that the patient has a chronic brain syndrome the social worker can be instrumental in helping to either support the family in caring for such a patient at home or where this is not possible, to assist in making arrangements for care in a skilled nursing facility.

Working with the patient and family to accept change in functioning, whether physical or mental, is important when planning for discharge. Another major part of discharge planning is helping to create alternatives for the older person and his or her family, as well as providing assistance in weighing the alternatives. The social worker must draw on the strengths available within the patient and family and attempt to create ways to provide supports for the deficits.

The family which will be caring for the demented individual at home following hospitalization may be helped by referral for the patient to day hospital programs where they exist, for extra help in the home to give the caregivers some respite, for participation in group programs for patients or families. The social worker may be able to help the family receive necessary information from their physician about the patient's condition. It is important not to allow hospital care to end with the diagnosis. Rather, assistance with further planning must be offered.

There are often situations in which the demented patient has no family or supportive network and the social worker may need to take an even more active role in planning for the patient.

Mrs. S., 77-years-old, was brought to the hospital because of confusion, disorientation, memory deficits, and inability to care for herself. She was admitted to the psychiatry unit of a general hospital.

Mrs. S. had intact social graces which initially made her appear quite able. However, extended conversation revealed major cognitive deficits. Her history was a mystery. No one came forward who had any knowledge of her outside the hospital. Her identification cards gave only her name and address.

While medical workup proceeded, the social worker tried to get information about how Mrs. S. had managed to cope until that point, given her very severe deficit. In the hope of obtaining more information and because Mrs. S. had grave concerns about some money left at her home, the social worker arranged with the nurse to accompany Mrs. S. to her home on a pass.

While at the hospital Mrs. S. was unable to find her own room or to remember the person she had held a conversation with 5 minutes before. It was striking to see her pull herself together when they arrived at her apartment building. Mrs. S. greeted the doorman, held her head high and led the way around the corner to the elevators. She greeted a gentleman in the elevator appropriately, asked about his wife and found her own apartment at the end of the hall. She confided to the social worker that she was "fooling" the people she had seen. They did not seem to be aware of how forgetful she really was, or that she was in fact a patient in the hospital.

The ability to be socially appropriate had helped to maintain Mrs. S. even as her mental capacities were failing. The apartment showed signs of having been kept up by someone, just as Mrs. S.'s well-dyed hair and polished nails on admission had been evidence of her having recently been to a beautician. Mrs. S. began to look for money and checkbooks she had hidden and despite rummaging and some anguish, she found what she had been seeking. The nurse and social worker found papers for Mrs. S. and learned the name of a lawyer who was taking care of her affairs.

The enormous difficulty Mrs. S had in functioning and her lack of sound judgment in many areas was only partially balanced by her social skills and the discovery of the lawyer-friend who had helped her periodically. Mrs. S. was a widow with no family and had apparently managed with very sporadic help from neighbors and weekly visits from the lawyer-friend.

Despite attempts at trying to create further community supports, Mrs. S. was too deteriorated to manage without constant supervision and eventually was transferred to a nursing home.

This example points up the necessity of flexibility in activities under the rubric of discharge in obtaining information and planning when the patient is confused and no ready relative stands by. Such are frequently concomitants of gerontological social work in the hospital.

Also inherent in working with older patients on discharge is the phenomenon of "paper work." In this setting the social worker frequently provides a major coordinating role. As a part of this endeavor written communications of various sorts are mandatory. Chart notes for formal communication with medical staff must be concise and informative. Letters to outside agencies or helpers need to spell out clearly what the needs of the patient are and the agreed service conditions.

Forms to be completed seem to accompany almost any request for service, benefit or change. It is nearly always part of the social worker's role to be responsible for the completion of such forms. This is frequently a time-consuming and frustrating task whether it involves checking off boxes which do not seem to fit what one really has to communicate, or tracking down other staff who must be asked to complete forms they are required to sign. In the latter situation, the social worker may often bear the brunt of others' frustrations about completing forms. The difficulties of this task, however, have not yet made it obsolete. Therefore, the responsiblity for using the paper flow most advantageously for the patient remains an important function of the social worker.

No discussion of social work in discharge planning would be complete without some mention of the patient who in hospital jargon becomes a "disposition problem." Such a person is usually old, generally very disabled physically and/or mentally, and needing large amounts of nursing care. Compounding his/her difficulties may be his/her financial level which places him/her just above the Medicaid eligibility levels but is insufficient to meet the high cost of nursing home care. This person needs residence and care in a skilled nursing facility, but because of bed shortages Homes can choose other "easier to care for" patients before admitting him/her. What occurs is that the patient will remain hospitalized much beyond the time he/she is medically ready to leave.

Such overstays have consequences for the patient, family and staff. The social worker not only has a major role in trying to facilitate placement but must work with patient and family around the prolonged uncertainty. Staff will have many reactions to the patient who presents "disposition problems," from "adopting" and protecting that patient, to angrily ignoring him or her. The "problem" is often seen as a failure of the social worker to effect a transfer of the patient.

In such instances, the social worker, while proceeding with the mechanics of effecting the transfer, must be active with the patient and family and work at interpreting the real situation to other staff.

3. Educating Other Hospital Staff

The hospital social worker shares information with other professionals about patients to contribute to the understanding and care of each individual. When dealing with the older patient the worker also needs to be knowledgeable about and able to communicate information regarding psychosocial issues in late life.

Developmental tasks of late life need to be understood and how they impact on the hospitalized elderly discussed. Often hospital staff are reluctant to take time necessary to really understand the older patient. Often they fear they will be recipients of irrelevant tales of the past. Social workers are generally more experienced with the use of reminis-cence as a therapeutic modality[17] but physicians and nurses can be helped to see the usefulness of reminiscence in their own work. They can be shown how they can understand a patient better and learn more about his or her prior health habits and coping styles. They can see how reminiscence about areas of interest to the patient can lead to establishing better rapport and that much history, important to diagnosis and treatment, can be elicited from the older patient. The social worker can also educate other staff regarding the therapeutic use of reminiscence in helping the older person gain strength from remembering "better days."

The social worker can be in the position of dispelling myths about the aged, both by referring to the literature in this area, and by pointing out the individuality of each patient.

The social worker can help staff balance a view of the acutely ill elderly patient they are seeing, with information on the heterogeneous nature of people within this population group. Often the social worker is able to use information about demographics, patterns, and trends to enrich the case by case experience of hospital staff.

While it is the social worker who is generally most active in helping older people obtain and manage their entitlements, information in this area must be shared with other staff. When physicians prescribe specific types of care, they need to know how the costs of these are covered. The social worker can provide education about the uses of Medicare, Medicaid, and can be instrumental in dispelling the myth that "older people have no financial worries in obtaining health care."

Most hospital staff have a need to learn the rationale behind the forms they are asked to help complete. The social worker must understand these forms and be able to explain their use to other staff. The worker's experience with how such forms are received and interpreted is gained through his or her contacts with personnel at outside agencies. Educating other staff around such issues can take place on a case by case basis, or even in small meetings held specifically for this purpose.

Another way to educate others is to be a role model. The way the social worker responds to the older patient and/or his family helps to set a tone for others. Social work values of autonomy and self-determination when applied to the older patient, are often a model for other staff to follow. Specific techniques for interviewing where there may be sensory impairment should be used. Some of these include attempting to cut out distractions when speaking to the older person. Another is having the worker face the older patient and take care that light is on his or her own face to aid the patient in comprehending. The social worker can demonstrate the use of touch where appropriate and should be skilled in assessing the mental status of any patient who may have some confusion. For the patient who does exhibit signs of dementia, the social worker must help staff see that the diagnosis alone, does not determine functioning, but that multiple variables exist and some of these may be amenable to change.

The social worker operates from the perspective of "person environment fit" as explicated by Coulton.[18] This refers to the "degree of congruence between an individual's needs, capacities and aspirations, and his environment's resource demands and opportunities." The worker is in the unique position of viewing the strengths and disabilities of the older person within the context of the environment in which he will need to function. This perspective can be shared with other staff and is helpful to each discipline involved in caring for the older patient.

4. Providing Support for Other Staff

Working with older people in the hospital can be a demanding task. It is emotionally draining to be faced with illness, frailty, and vulnerability, as well as to deal with people often in a precarious balance of interacting deficits. Older patients frequently present complex diagnostic problems and complicated social situations. In the acute hospital pressures are high, the pace rapid, but the older patient frequently needs more time and greater patience than younger patients.

Hospital staff need support in the giving of skilled, compassionate care to elderly patients. They need help in seeing the challenges of giving such care. The hospital system does not have built-in rewards for this. Social work is one discipline which can take on a supportive role in this area.

> Mrs. R., a quiet 69-year-old Hispanic woman, came to the hospital with shortness of breath, malnutrition, and some confusion. She had been living alone in a small apartment prior to admission. With treatment, she improved past her medical crisis and was gaining strength and stability. She asked for nothing, seemed appreciative of any attention shown her, but was content to lie in her bed and initiate no activity.
>
> Ms. S., the R.N. assigned to her care, realized that Mrs. R. needed more stimulation, encouragement, and assistance in walking and in making her wishes known. Ms. S. took extra time to talk to Mrs. R., to bring her the extra coffee she began to ask for, and to initiate a regimen of assisting her in walking more each day to regain the use of her limbs. The social worker was active with Mrs. R. in planning to have a home attendant help the patient when she returned home. The social worker also provided encouragement and support for Ms. S.'s efforts with the patient and gave the nurse direct recognition at staff meetings for her major role in motivating Mrs. R. During setbacks which occurred in the

patient's progress, the social worker continued to be supportive to the nurse. All of this reinforced Ms. S.'s motivation and supported her work with the patient.

The social worker can help a staff member to understand his or her own reactions to a particular older patient, can listen to frustrations and misgivings, can encourage the giving of time and energy to older patients. All these activities enter into the support the social worker can provide to those who deal with older patients.

Social work as a profession brings to the hospital setting a respect for the need to collaborate, and skills in engaging various others to participate together. These are essential in working toward optimal care for the older patient. The expertise in human development, systems negotiation, and resource management that social workers have is helpful not only for the patients, but is supportive for other staff as well.

Summary

Gerontological social work in the acute hospital is an amalgam of the best that is in us. We are dealing with a vulnerable group at point of crises, and are instrumental in providing understanding and services necessary to the continued functioning of that person.

In the acute care hospital, the social worker is engaged in direct service to the older patient and his or her family, in collaborative work with other professionals, in negotiating the hospital system and in bridging the gap between the outside community and the institution. In order to do all this effectively, the worker must have a secure sense of his or her own professional identity. He or she must be flexible, creative and strong in the face of numerous and often conflicting pressures.

Working with older people on an outpatient basis demands the same qualities and practices that have been discussed. The primary care role for such outpatients also demands the same comprehensive assessments and interventive strategies to support strengths, shore up deficits and prevent breakdown.

It is impossible to cover every function of social work with older people in the hospital, but it is important to realize the complexity and challenges involved. Above all the acute care hospital must be seen as part of the overall care available to older persons. It is a major function of social work to place the acute care hospital squarely within the continuum of long-term care.

REFERENCES

1. Shanas, Ethel & Maddox, George. "Aging, Health and Organization of Health Resources," *Handbook of Aging and the Social Sciences*, Ed. by Robert Binstock and Ethel Shanas. New York: Van Nostrand Reinhold & Co., 1976, p. 593.

2. U.S. Department of Health, *Health, U.S. 1975* Public Health Service, Health Research Administration Department of Health, Education & Welfare Publication Number (HRA) 76-1232, Washington, D.C.: Government Printing Office, p. 513, 573.

3. Pegels, C. Carl. *Health Care and the Elderly*, Rockville, MD: Aspen Systems Corporation, 1980, p. 5.

4. Knowles, John H. "The Hospital," *Scientific American*, 229, September, 1973 p. 128

5. Ibid, p. 132

6. Blumenfield, Susan. *Counselor-Assistants for a Geriatric Program in a Community Hospital*, City University of New York: unpublished doctoral thesis, 1977, p. 15.

7. Mauksch, Hans O. "The Organizational Context of Dying," *Death: The Final Stage of Growth*, Ed. by Elisabeth Kubler-Ross. Englewood Cliffs, NJ: Prentice-Hall, Inc., 1975, p.15.

8. Ibid, p.19

9. Engel, George L. "The Clinical Application of the Biopsychosocial Model." *The American Journal of Psychiatry*, May 1980, pp. 535-543.

10. Berkman, B. & Rehr, H. "Social Needs of the Hospitalized Elderly: A Classification." *Social Work*, July 1972, pp. 80-88.

11. Erikson, Erik. *Childhood and Society*, New York: W.W. Norton & Company, Inc. 1963.

12. Butler, Robert. *Why Survive? Being Old in America*, New York, Harper & Row Publishers, 1975.

13. Libow, L. & Sherman, F. *The Core of Geriatric Medicine*, St. Louis: C.V. Mosby, Co., 1981.

14. Saul, Shura. *Aging: An Album of People Growing Old*, New York: John Wiley and Sons, Inc., 1974.

15. Monk, Abraham, "Social Work with the Aged: Principles of Practice." *Social Work*, January 1981, pp. 61-68.

16. Kastenbaum, Robert. "Reluctant Therapist." In *New Thoughts on Old Age*, Ed. Robert Kastenbaum, New York: Springer Publishing Co., 1964 pp. 139-145.

17. Pincus, Allen. "Reminiscence in Aging & Its Implications for Social Work Practice." *Social Work*, July 1970, Vol. 15, pp. 47-53.

18. Coulton, Claudia. "A Study of Person-Environment Fit Among the Chronically Ill". *Social Work in Health Care*, Vol. 5, No. 1. Fall 1979.

Chapter 3

MAXIMIZING INDEPENDENCE
FOR THE ELDERLY:
THE SOCIAL WORKER
IN THE REHABILITATION CENTER

Gary B. Seltzer
Marcel O. Charpentier

Introduction

As we become more of an aging society, with the number of older persons expected to double by the year 2030, the need to maintain maximum functional independence and productivity in this segment of the population increases. The provision of rehabilitation services, particularly at points of crisis, is an essential component of a responsive long-term care system which attempts to divert high risk elders away from institutional care toward less restrictive alternatives. The practices of rehabilitation medicine target maintenance of functioning as a primary intervention goal—moving beyond the prototypic stress on curing to a treatment emphasis based on how a person performs activities of daily living in spite of the presence of chronic disease and physical impairments. The elderly are particularly vulnerable to limitations in essential activities, with those age 75 years and older twenty times more likely than the under 75 age group to have limitations in at least one of the following four personal care activity areas: bathing, dressing, eating, and toileting.[1]

As a rule, older persons with functional limitations and serious chronic conditions are cared for by their families. It is estimated that families and friends give between 60 to 80% of the care received by functionally limited elderly persons.[2] Families tend to provide this care usually without compensation and until a crisis stage arises. The types of crises typically encountered include such occurrences as onset of a new acute medical problem, further deterioration of functioning, or increased intrafamilial emotional problems. Oftentimes, it is at these crisis points that a short-term rehabilitation treatment intervention can be helpful in restoring a sufficient level of functioning to the elderly person and to the informal support system. Anticipated outcomes of such an intervention might be to prevent institutional placement, to reduce the length of stay if institutionalization is necessary, or to facilitate placement in a residential setting that is less restrictive than a nursing home (e.g., a domiciliary care home).

The role of social work practice within an acute rehabilitation setting is the focus of this chapter. The case examples and some setting dynamics are drawn from the Rehabilitation Unit at The Memorial Hospital, Pawtucket, Rhode Island, a Brown University affiliated teaching hospital. Although we have chosen to highlight this setting, we have not limited ourselves to the type of social work practice that occurs on this unit. Instead, we describe practice principles that are applicable to a variety of short-term medical rehabilitation settings that treat older, functionally impaired persons. Furthermore, our discussion of social work treatment interventions and anticipated outcomes is relevant to the broader service context of the long-term care system.

Evaluation of Rehabilitation Potential

The rationale for a patient's acceptance into or rejection from the Rehabilitation Unit is often explained to families and third party payers on the basis of the patient's estimated rehabilitation potential. Since rehabilitation personnel use the construct of "rehabilitation potential" to guide entry decisions, length of stay, and discharge determinations, the conceptual and operational definition of this construct must be examined. In particular, the type of assessment approach and conceptual underpinnings employed in making a judgment about a patient's rehabilitation potential are discussed below. The social worker needs a thorough understanding of the construct "rehabilitation potential" because he or she often assumes responsibility for communicating to the elderly patient and his/her family the rehabilitation team's findings regarding the patient's rehabilitation potential.

The concept "rehabilitation potential" has three possible meanings. First, it implies that functions (such as walking) which were lost as a result of physical and/or psychological problems may be restored through rehabilitation. Second, rehabilitation potential suggests that, in addition to restoring lost functions, the patient has latent capabilities (e.g., a right-handed patient learning to write with his/her left hand after having a left hemispheric stroke) which, when treated during rehabilitation, will become manifest. Third, rehabilitation potential implies that the deterioration in functioning experienced by some patients can be slowed down. This definition of rehabilitation potential stresses the potential for rehabilitation to result in no change in functioning (maintenance) or the slowing down of functional decline when the absence of rehabilitation treatment would be expected to result in more rapid decline in functioning.

Brody stresses the importance of the latter meaning of rehabilitation potential when therapeutic interventions are being designed for the so-called "frail elderly":

> . . . it cannot be assumed that the slope of decline is so inevitable that one becomes therapeutically nihilistic. The goals are (1) to identify and reduce "excess disabilities" that are imposed by environments or by lack of care—that is to close the gap between actual functioning and potential functioning, taking nothing for granted and (2) to meet residual dependencies in such a way as to promote independence and well being. . . . The word *potential* is key for realistic goals with frail elderly including maintenance of function and retardation of decline as well as improvement.

Since this third definition of rehabilitation potential runs counter to the traditional connotation of rehabilitation as only restorative care, elderly patients who might benefit from an intervention aimed at slowing down the debilitating effects of a chronic health problem are too rarely referred for an assessment of their potential.

The assessment of rehabilitation potential focuses on a determination of the consequences of physical and psychosocial impairments by means of an examination of the specific kinds of activities in which a person can or cannot engage. In addition, as Brody noted, it is important to evaluate the environmental and social conditions which facilitate or pose obstacles to patients in their performance of activities. The types of functional activities assessed typically include, but are not limited to, the following:

1. personal activities of daily living or personal care tasks, such as bowel and bladder continence, mobility, and self care;
2. instrumental activities of daily living, such as shopping, household repairs, and telephoning;

3. leisure time activities, such as reading, hobbies, and attending social events;
4. sexual functioning;
5. vocational or educational activities;
6. mental status and other psychological functions;
7. interactions within formal and informal support systems.

These areas are assessed because they are important to a person's independence and quality of life. Assessing the person's behavioral strengths and weaknesses and their environmental supports and barriers provide the critical data necessary for an analysis of how prospective rehabilitation patients are likely to cope with their physical and social limitations after a rehabilitation intervention. Once the assessment data are collected on the above delineated areas, an analysis is made of a person's functional level. According to Granger, "Analysis of function means identification and classification of functional abilities and functional limitations. A functional limitation is a consequence of a health problem and represents an inability to meet a standard of expectation; thus, the concept incorporates deficits of an anatomical, physiological, psychological or mental nature (impairment), deficits in the behavioral performance of skills and tasks (disability) or deficits in fulfillment of social roles (handicap)."[4]

The intent of analyzing function in this model is to go beyond the traditional "medical model" which tends to delimit its purview to the characteristics of disease.[5] When analyzing for rehabilitation potential an examination should be made of the disabilities and handicaps that result from disease along with an appropriate evaluation of the medical aspects of the disease. The following case example is presented in order to further illustrate the assessment and analysis of rehabilitation potential.

Case Illustration: Mrs. R.

Mrs. R. is a 79-year-old woman, who five years prior to rehabilitation assessment consultation had had a stroke which resulted in a left hemiparesis. She was discharged from the hospital after her stroke and did not enter into a rehabilitation unit. She did receive physical therapy for a few months and learned to walk with a walker. She and her family expected more return in her upper limb which did not occur. Until his sudden death two months prior to the consultation, Mrs. R. lived with her husband in a second-floor apartment. She was dependent upon him for shopping, cooking, and some self-care activities. Her two children, a son and a daughter, had supplemented their father's care of Mrs. R. but had not assumed primary responsibility. At the time of the consultation, Mrs. R. was alternately living with each of her children and their families. Her children, although supportive, did not feel it was possible for Mrs. R. to remain living with either of them.

The rehabilitation potential assessment focused on the question of whether it would be possible to restore sufficient functional abilities in order for Mrs. R. to live independently and not be placed in a long-term care facility. Her functional limitations consequent to her stroke and minimal previous rehabilitation training were in the areas of mobility and upper limb functional tasks such as self care and instrumental activities of daily living (e.g., cooking and cleaning). According to the above analytic schema, Mrs. R.'s impairments were in her upper and lower limbs and the disabilities were in her lack of performance of daily tasks necessary for fulfilling her expected social role of living independently.

The assessment of the extent of her handicap (i.e., ability to fulfill social roles) falls most often within the domain of the social worker. That is, if Mrs. R. has the potential to cope at some level with her disabilities after a rehabilitation intervention, can she be helped to adapt to her handicap? In this case, can Mrs. R. learn to live on her own with the support of her family and the support of community services?

After assessing Mrs. R. it was felt that with the receipt of intensive occupational therapy to compensate for her upper limb dysfunction and physical therapy to increase her mobility, Mrs. R. could perform more of the tasks necessary for independent living than she presently performed. Furthermore, it was felt that her family support could be structured to supplement her care needs along with community services such as adapted elderly housing and homemaker services. Mrs. R. was then admitted to the rehabilitation unit to implement the plan derived from the assessment and analysis of her rehabilitation potential.

The Practice Framework

The average length of stay on The Memorial Hospital Rehabilitation Unit is three to four weeks; patients rarely remain for more than six weeks. The most common presenting medical problems are stroke and amputation, although a fair number of patients are also accepted for other neurological and musculoskeletal problems. A criterion for admission to the unit is that the patients are no longer in need of acute medical care;

however, frequently patients are admitted who require medical management for such problems as hypertension, diabetes, or cardiopulmonary insufficiency. Often, patients arrive on the unit immediately following the acute phase of their illness and may not have begun an emotional adjustment to the extent to which they are limited in performing routine daily activities such as dressing, bathing, and grooming. To complicate matters, most patients are admitted from acute care medical-surgical units where they are expected to play the "patient role" and not perform self care activities. Thus, many patients are facing the behavioral and emotional consequences of their illnesses for the first time when they enter the Rehabilitation Unit. At this point in time, patients and family are often experiencing an acute reaction to what is likely to be a chronic problem.

Since length of stay on the unit is time-limited, the patient and family need to simultaneously maintain sufficient equilibrium to work through their emotional reactions to the physical limitation and commit themselves to the stressful process of restoring as much physical functioning as is possible. Thus, the time to intervene is limited, the hazardous event is a significant loss in physical functioning, and the tasks to be accomplished are usually emotionally stressful and physically exhausting. In light of these demands on patients and families, the model of social work practice on this unit is based upon crisis theory. As Rapoport notes, "Crisis theory explicitly refrains from defining or equating the state of crisis with an illness . . . we need to abandon the concept of cure and shift to the concept of restoration and enhancement of functioning."[6] The focus for the patient and social worker on the rehabilitation unit is on the restoration of optimal functioning in spite of pathological conditions which are unlikely to be reversed. To help the client and family accomplish this task of restoring optimal functioning, the social worker needs to employ techniques such as those suggested by Parad, "direct advice, encouragement of adaptive behavior, anticipatory guidance, and environmental manipulation.[7] In particular, clients need to learn a new or supplemental behavioral repertoire to compensate for their physical, social, and emotional losses. Therefore, it is essential for the worker to know that "the goal in crisis brief treatment is action and furtherance of rapid behavior change with positive reinforcement."[8]

The social worker is in a unique position to use positive reinforcement contingently with the patient and family. Among all the rehabilitation team members, the social worker typically emerges as the person responsible for helping to provide service linkages both during the hospital stay and upon release. If the social worker begins discharge planning when patients are admitted (as we suggest in more detail later in the chapter), he/she can be perceived as a reinforcing and trusting agent through which the patient and family system can resolve present and future problems. For example, the social worker can help the client and family understand the team's treatment goals and medical aspects of the situation. In this way, the social worker has an instrumental role in helping to clarify and direct the client system toward understanding, accepting and planning reasonable rehabilitation treatment outcomes.

The following case study describes the social worker's role in delineating and negotiating with client systems those strategic tasks which lead to a successful course of rehabilitation.

Case Illustration: Mrs. K.

Mrs. K. is an 82-year-old woman, with severe osteoporosis (a degenerative bone disease), and chronic lower back pain. Two days prior to her hospital admission she was attempting to open a window, heard a snap, and felt a sharp pain in her back. On admission she was unable to walk without excruciating pain. X-rays revealed a compression fracture. After four days of bedrest and pain medication she was referred for evaluation of rehabilitation potential.

Mrs. K. had been living with her daughter and her family since her husband's death. Upon his death some four years ago, Mrs. K. moved from Florida where she and her husband had lived for fifteen years after his retirement. In Florida, she and her husband had had an active social life. Dancing had been one of the couple's favorite activities. Since moving North to live with her daughter, Mrs. K.'s social life centered solely around her daughter's family. Mrs. K.'s daughter was employed and her children attended school, leaving Mrs. K. alone most of the day. When she was able to, Mrs. K. spent her time performing cleaning chores. With the increasing pain she was less able to perform these activities and had begun to increasingly focus on her pain.

When the social worker interviewed Mrs. K. and her daughter their relationship appeared strained and both expressed a sense of urgency. Mrs. K.'s daughter, not knowing what her mother could or could not do, was planning to leave her job in order to care for her mother. In describing her plans, it was clear that she intended to care for her mother by restricting her mother's activities. Mrs. K., who already was expressing feelings of being useless, did not want to be further restricted but also did not want to risk thwarting her daughter's intentions lest it result in her losing the attention and care she needed.

In fact, Mrs. K. had learned to control her daughter's attention with her reports of pain. The social worker had a limited amount of time to advise Mrs. K. and her daughter about the levels of activities that might reduce the social and emotional losses for both. First, Mrs. K.'s daughter needed to be instructed to observe her mother during rehabilitation activities such as physical therapy so she could learn that her mother could mobilize herself in spite of pain. She needed to learn when to ignore the pain and when to encourage her mother to complete an activity rather than prevent the activity from occurring. Second, the social worker had to guide the mother and daughter into accepting the need for Mrs. K. to extend her social activities beyond the immediate family. Third, the social worker encouraged both the mother and daughter to contract for engaging in household activities which Mrs. K. could do with minimum risks to herself yet gave her a sense of being useful.

The social worker began the treatment intervention when Mrs. K. entered the unit and upon discharge had completed all of the above delineated tasks. The daughter remained employed, and Mrs. K. was scheduled to attend a Senior Citizens Center for a part of everyday. By structuring interactions between both parties while Mrs. K. was on the unit, the social worker was able to guide the clients toward the tasks which they had agreed to perform following Mrs. K.'s discharge home.

The preceding case illustration emphasizes the proactive social work tasks necessary to develop positive coping reactions within a family system. Appreciating the mutual needs of both mother and daughter, the social worker was able to help preserve a sense of independence for Mrs. K. while concurrently reducing the daughter's need to feel totally responsible for her mother's well-being. A combined focus upon (1) timely assessment and educational intervention, and (2) the mobilization of available informal supports, enabled the accomplishment of a variety of environmental/interactional changes culminating in discharge to the client's home rather than to an institutional setting.

The Experience of Rehabilitation

Ideally, social work intervention will already have been initiated prior to admission to the rehabilitation unit. If so, the existing social data base collected during a pre-admission assessment may be reviewed to determine the tasks necessary for engaging the client/family in active participation within a formalized rehabilitation program. In many situations, however, the sociomedical assessment of rehabilitation potential at the point of admission provides the first opportunity for both patient and family to benefit from casework intervention.

As noted earlier, casework intervention in this setting is heavily reliant upon crisis theory. The situational crisis of physical illness, as with non-physically induced crises, tends to follow a continuum of overlapping phases—onset, acute, recuperative, and restorative.[9] Typically, social work intervention occurs during the acute phase of active medical treatment or the recuperation phase, the latter phase of which strives toward the gradual recovery of pre-crisis functioning. Often, social work efforts during the acute phase of treatment sets the therapeutic stage for continued progress in the recuperation (or physical rehabilitation) phase.

In examining the social worker practice role unique to elderly persons undergoing rehabilitation treatment following acute physical illness, we shall emphasize the following five rehabilitation-specific factors: (1) the entry phase, (2) the team/client interface, (3) the interpretation of team assessment, (4) client adaptation, and (5) the social work role in assisting the client/family to deal with functional limitations.

The Entry Phase

The interim period between admission to the hospital and transfer to a rehabilitation program is one characterized by anxiety, uncertainty, and confusion engendered by entry into a new setting. It is during this turbulent period that the client and family must make difficult decisions affecting the outcome of illness. While submerged within an acutely distressful event, family members are, of necessity, requested to consider a perceived "distant" future as part of the team's effort to accurately assess the degree of potential socio-environmental support available following discharge At this juncture, it is difficult for significant others to adjust to their fears of excessive responsibility for the total physical care of the newly disabled person. These fears are based, in part, on the family's inability to recognize potential functional gains as well as their perception of the acute physical trauma as an unalterable end product. Compounding the family's feelings of insecurity are the limited community services available to older disabled family members, as well as realistic financial constraints endemic within the elderly population.

The Team/Client Interface

It is absolutely essential for team members to continually appreciate the non-professional community's lack of familiarity with many components of the rehabilitation process. The team's emphasis on independence as opposed to dependent nurturance, its daily exposure to illness and disability as the norm, its reliance upon both empirical and experiential knowledge in assessment of rehabilitation potential, and its routine use of adaptive medical appliances are all situational components foreign to the typical client. These factors, compounded by pre-existent "hidden agendas" in family interaction, combine to make the relatively brief encounter within a rehabilitation program a true challenge to both the client system's adaptive abilities and the teams's successful application of its collective expertise. Given these circumstances, it is incumbent upon the social worker to develop an effective communication linkage between the client system and the professional staff.

Interpretation of Team Assessment

Once the initial interdisciplinary team evaluation has been completed following transfer to the unit, a prescheduled patient/family conference is often utilized as a forum to further clarify components of the rehabilitation process. This additional encounter has been recognized as a valuable means of allaying anxiety.[10] Key team members involved with the patient, as well as significant others, may serve as participants. Content should include explanations to the patient and family of the distinct functions and roles of relevant team disciplines (physical therapy, social work, medicine, speech therapy, psychology, etc.); major life areas which typically require psychological and/or environmental readjustments (lost roles, altered relationships, adaptive devices, housing, etc.); and broader concerns such as realistic goals attainable during time-limited rehabilitation, adaptation to society's view of disability/handicap, and reintegration into the community.

The above informational exchange serves as both a springboard to participation as well as a demonstration of the cooperative nature of this complicated task. Again, team members must be sensitive to the client/family's ability (or inability) to integrate—and act upon—the available information. A continuum of emotional reactions, ranging from complete acceptance of functional limitations to fantasies about total recovery, will heavily affect how objective data will be interpreted.

Client Adaptation

As a participant within the rehabilitation program, the patient must undergo significant readjustments in order to ensure successful treatment. The most outstanding of these changes involves the daily regimen of hospital care. Unlike the acute medical phase of treatment during which the patient is encouraged to remain dependent and inactive, the emphasis during rehabilitation is upon efforts directed toward as high a level of participation and initiative as is possible for each patient. Daily tasks of bathing, toileting, eating, dressing, and mobility become the responsibility of the patient—not his/her hospital caretakers. Throughout this gradual progression from dependence to self-sufficiency, the patient is educated to perform necessary tasks within the constraints imposed by incapacitating impairments. The resultant increase in psychological/physical independence tends to enhance self-image, self-confidence, and self-respect, ultimately leading to a frame of reference conducive to long-term retention of previously defined goals.

Social Work Role

Throughout the entry process, it is incumbent upon the social worker to be consistently available in order to provide the diversity of services required to assist families in crisis. In addition to ensuring access to basic environmental support services, the social worker must utilize the helping relationship as a mechanism wherein the various implications of functional limitations may be addressed. Issues such as altered self-image, changed lifestyle, decreased generativity, reduced energy level, increased dependency, role reversal, and negative outlook on life must be openly discussed and examined. This approach increases the likelihood of developing positive family/patient coping patterns during recuperation and restoration.

The responsibility for addressing these issues, although shared among many team members throughout the treatment process, remains primarily that of the social worker. As the professional trained to assist the patient/ family alter their attitudes and resolve emotional problems, the social worker provides directed support in the area of effective re-education. Traditional casework techniques such as facilitating emotive expression, legitimizing grief reactions associated with loss of bodily function, and utilizing subjective elements within the helping relationship must be combined with an objectively planned approach of teaching the client/family new coping strategies and/or patterns of communication.

The Discharge Planning Process

Discharge planning is generally defined as the social work activity which helps patients to: (1) cope with hospitalization, (2) cope with illness and its effects, (3) move through the health care system, and (4) return to the community with appropriate supports.[11] In the interdisciplinary rehabilitation setting, the social worker acts as the central coordinator for each team member's contribution to the discharge plan, while simultaneously performing a linkage role between hospital-based services and community-based support networks activated following discharge.[12] In order for the social worker to coordinate the discharge planning effort effectively, he/she must be able to understand the terminology peculiar to each discipline and know many of the clinical aspects of each discipline's assessment and treatment procedures. Having the ability to understand this interdisciplinary knowledge, the social worker can initiate discharge planning upon a patient's admission to the rehabilitation unit and thereby achieve the above delineated discharge planning activities.

If the rehabilitation unit utilizes a quantitative functional assessment to measure a patient's physical functioning, then the social worker has some key data available with which to design a discharge plan. As noted earlier, rehabilitation treatment focuses on the restoration, maintenance, or slowing down of deterioration of physical functions such as dressing, grooming, bladder and bowel continence, transferring, walking, etc. A functional assessment instrument which has been used extensively in medical rehabilitation is the Barthel Index as modified by Granger.[13] The Barthel Index measures the degree to which a patient can perform independently activities of daily living (e.g., self care, transfer to toilet, walking 50 yards, etc.). Essentially, the Barthel Index measures the degree of severity of a patient's physical handicap, a measurement which has been shown to be highly related to discharge placement—home versus long-term care facilities,[14] and to the number of hours and service needs for long-term care in the home setting.[15]

Using the Barthel Index or some other measure of physical functioning, the social worker can predict the level of function that is likely to be restored during hospitalization and the physical limitations that are likely to remain upon a patient's discharge. For example, if it is known that a patient is likely to be continent upon discharge and able to get to a toilet or commode with no more than minimal assistance but still has trouble walking, and has difficulty with some dressing skills, then the social worker knows that the patient is likely to require about two hours of daily help from significant others. Armed with this very specific type of information, the social worker can help the patient and his/her family maintain appropriate expectations for the tasks to be accomplished during the hospital stay and the types of service plans and familial supports necessary upon discharge.

In addition to using the functional assessment data collected by other rehabilitation team members, the social worker is responsible for assessing the patient's psychological and social functioning. According to Hollis, a psychosocial study may be defined as "the process of observation and classification of the facts observed about a client and his/her situation, with the purpose of securing as much information as is needed to understand the client and his/her problem and to guide treatment wisely."[16] As a result of the time-limited and crisis oriented context within which this assessment is completed, the social worker gives particular attention to the rehabilitation continuum (health-illness-impairment) as it affects the client/family constellation. The social worker must clearly identify the unique psychosocial stresses impinging upon older patients.[17] And, as part of the assessment process, the social worker should conduct interviews with an elderly spouse, siblings, adult children, extended family members or close friends. The enlistment of this natural helping network becomes an essential step in increasing the likelihood of a successful return to the community.[18]

An integral component of the discharge planning process on a rehabilitating unit is the completion of at least one therapeutic home visit (THV). The patient's home should be either accessible in terms of mobility and daily living tasks, or have the potential to be appropriately modified. Also, during the THV, a significant other person must be available to supervise the patient at home and function as a caretaker when necessary. The THV is accomplished as soon as the patient is deemed medically stable enough to endure several hours of supervised activity in his/her home. The THV has the following goals: (1) to provide a realistic experience for both patient and family of potential problem areas prior to discharge, (2) to alert hospital staff of potential needs which can be met through referral to community support agencies, and (3) to develop a plan of action to rectify structural obstacles in areas of accessibility and mobility. (See Figure I). The THV should assess the need for communication aids, personal care equipment, mobility aids, housing modifications, and formal community supports. Once completed, the available data are employed by members of the rehabilitation team to create an individualized discharge plan for each patient.

Figure 1. Items Assessed During Therapeutic Home Visit

DO YOU NEED:	COMMUNICATION AIDS	YES
1) Hearing aid		( )
2) Telephone or telephone adaptation		( )
3) Call alarm system		( )

PERSONAL CARE EQUIPMENT

*4) Aids for dressing (stocking assist, long shoehorn, button hook)		( )
*5) Aids for reaching		( )
*6) Aids for feeding (rocker knife, plate guard)		( )
*7) Special clothing		( )
*8) Special shoes		( )
*9) Elastic stocking		( )
10) Brace or corset		( )
11) Arm sling or arm roll		( )
12) Prosthetic limb		( )
13) Bedpan		( )
14) Urinal		( )
15) Catheters, collecting bags for bladder, etc.		( )
16) Fitted bowel appliances, including ostomy, etc.		( )
17) Absorbent pads		( )
18) Waterproof bedding		( )
19) Waterproof clothing		( )

MOBILITY AIDS

20) Crutches, cane, walker, etc.		( )
21) Wheelchair or wheelchair accessories (cushion)		( )
*22) Toilet grab bars		( )
*23) Raised toilet seat		( )
*24) Shower seat		( )
25) Bedside commode		( )
26) Hospital bed		( )
*27) Transfer belt		( )

*These items are not generally covered by Medicare/Medicaid or Blue Cross. Others may or may not be covered depending upon your disability and/or type of insurance.

HOUSING MODIFICATIONS**

28) Ramps or rails inside or outside the house		( )
29) Special handles or switches		( )
30) A lift between floor levels		( )
31) A special bed to chair transfer device		( )
32) Bathroom modifications		( )
33) Bedroom modifications		( )
34) Kitchen modifications		( )

**Modifications are not made by the hospital but rehab staff will be glad to advise you on specifications.

ADVICE ON

35) Financial benefits		( )
36) Community services		( )
37) Health and social services		( )
38) Aids and equipment		( )
39) Transportation		( )

*** OTHER NEEDS?

As a rule, an important portion of the individualized discharge plan includes the service matrix needed by the patient and his/her family. In general, three categories of possible formal support systems exist in the service matrix: (1) those meeting concrete needs, (2) those providing medical/nursing care, and (3) those providing psychosocial/counselling services. The social worker's decision to refer a patient to one or more services is contingent upon the professional assessment of rehabilitation potential, as well as the needs expressed by the patient/family.

The first category, concrete services, includes housing, Senior Transportation, Homemaker Services, Meals on Wheels, or equipment suppliers. The second area, medical/nursing services, is provided through local Visiting Nurse Associations, a Coordinated Hospital Based Homecare Program, regular outpatient therapies (speech, occupational, or physical), etc. For those patients with identified mental health needs, a referral to a mental health center, family service agency, disease-specific peer support group (Alcoholics Anonymous, Stroke Club, Parkinson's Association, etc.), or Telephone Assurance Program may be indicated to preserve gains accomplished during inpatient treatment. Finally, some community-based agencies capable of providing multiple services in a centralized setting—a Senior Citizens's Center, the Division of Vocational Rehabilitation, the Paraplegia Association, or Community Action Program, may be called upon to assist during the post-rehabilitation phase. Whatever combination of services is deemed necessary, the existence of an individualized discharge service plan is a necessary component in assuring continuity of care for each discipline involved.

The following case example illustrates factors associated with functional impairment and the implementation of discharge planning services. The psychosocial struggles imposed upon the client system are highlighted as well as the role which emotional reactions play in determining rehabilitation outcome.

Case Illustration: Mr. L.

Mr. L., a 69-year-old, married white male of Canadian-American descent, was stricken while at work with sudden left-sided flaccidness of both extremities and slight aphasia. During the initial period of acute hospitalization, Mr. L. also suffered a moderate myocardial infarction, thereby prolonging the period between the acute onset of disabling illness and the initiation of intensive rehabilitation. Due to medical, financial, and behavioral complications, social work intervention had been initiated prior to Mr. L.'s arrival on the rehabilitation unit.

Interviews with Mr. and Mrs. L. revealed the following social data. Both Mr. and Mrs. L. were employed full-time—Mr. L. as a purchasing agent at an industrial firm, and Mrs. L. as a receptionist at a manufacturing plant. The L.'s were married 34 years, owned their own home, and had three adult children living independently. Characteristically, the L.'s were an industrious couple, with Mr. L. a leader within his social community. This sudden illness represented the first of its kind to occur among immediate family members.

Initially, Mr. L. remained extremely depressed, with sporadic verbalizations concentrating mainly on loss of functioning, fear of lost employment, financial catastrophe, and a slow rate of recovery. This predictable reaction was complicated by various cognitive/perceptual distortions induced by Mr. L.'s stroke. As physical gains were made during the following nine weeks, Mr. L.'s depressive affect was gradually transformed into an adaptive acceptance of his newly acquired self-image.

By the fourth week of rehabilitation, Mr. L. had regained his ability to ambulate with the assistance of a hemi-cane and limited support from another person. A therapeutic home visit was also accomplished during this week to determine necessary environmental alterations prior to discharge. However, Mr. L.'s persistent left-arm flaccidity, moderate urinary incontinence, and perceptual deficits remained primary obstacles to an independent return home. These issues were continually reassessed through daily social work intervention and several patient/family team conferences.

By the sixth week, both Mr. and Mrs. L. had reached the point of sheer exasperation due to continued left-arm flaccidity. Their reactions, especially those of Mrs. L., turned to anger directed against the perceived ineffective rehabilitation efforts. This ultimately resulted in attempts to obtain admission to a longer-term setting. These attempts represented this couple's inability to recognize the existence of a permanent functional deficit. Techniques of empathy, reality reinforcement, cognitive restructuring, and communication-skills enhancement eventually facilitated the L.'s integration of their altered lifestyle and expectations.

As anticipated discharge approached, and Mr. L. had developed sufficient self-confidence (tempered by realistic restraint), Mrs. L.'s fears and anxieties grew to maladaptive proportions. Despite Mrs. L.'s repeatedly expressed anger toward team members during the final phase prior to discharge, the social worker was able to maintain professional objectivity and served as both a "filter" for other team members and a source of consistent, nonjudgmental support to the L.'s. This use of relationship enabled Mrs. L. to express her deepest concerns, for the first time, in the presence of her husband during a structured interview.

Eventually, after nine weeks of involvement in the rehabilitation program (an unusually long stay necessitated by the medical complication of an acute myocardial infarction while hospitalized), Mr. L. was discharged home with the assistance of his wife, several friends, the local Visiting Nurse Service and Vocational Rehabilitation Agency, and various medical appliances.

The experience of Mr. L. clearly illustrates several aspects of the discharge planning process. The need for social work intervention shortly following hospital admission was accomplished through effective case screening to address initial financial concerns. This early interaction also enabled the formulation of a comprehensive psychosocial data base from which later rehabilitation potential factors could be considered. As rehabilitation progressed, anticipated environmental modifications were assessed through several therapeutic home visits. These visits provided invaluable data regarding structural changes necessary in the home in addition to highlighting further interactional problems which would likely affect implementation of the discharge plan. Finally, the directed use of a consistently available helping relationship allowed an element of trust to develop which in turn helped to offset the great degree of anxiety affecting implementation of final discharge arrangements.

Summary and Discussion

Within the next fifty years, the percentage of United States' residents age sixty-five or older will dramatically increase. It has therefore become imperative for the health care system's long-term care component to redirect its primary focus from one of basic maintenance to one of restoring or preserving functional independence. The provision of comprehensive rehabilitation services, encompassing both physical and psychosocial treatments, has proven to be an effective approach whereby older persons previously destined for institutional settings are returned home. A key factor in accomplishing this redirection is the enlistment of both formal and informal community support systems.

To some extent, the rehabilitation services described in this chapter can serve as a long-term care bridge between constricted choices typically available to an older person with severe physical impairments and other alternatives made possible when environmental, social, familial, psychological, and physical supports are activated to ensure maximum quality of life for the older person. Long-term care is usually represented by a variety of settings including extended care facilities, congregate living arrangements, or increased services in one's home. To the recipient, long-term care universally represents the existence of significant losses and subsequent restrictions. Many elders in need of long-term care must adapt to losses of money, physical abilities, personal autonomy, sensory activity, friendship ties, and family interaction. Yet, to maintain control of one's quality of life, an elder usually needs the opportunity to marshall supportive resources and thereby minimize the losses associated with feelings of hopelessness and helplessness. The intent of rehabilitation—to restore functional ability, to treat both the physical and psychosocial needs of the person, to gather resources, and to maximize independence can serve as an antidote to the onslaught of losses associated with long-term care.

The social worker is in the pivotal position among other rehabilitation specialists to understand and develop a plan of care which can influence the quality of life for elders with significant physical and/or cognitive impairments. By attending to practice principles described in this chapter, the social worker can assist the older person and his/her family to adjust to the severe demands imposed by physical limitations and associated emotional stressors.

REFERENCES

1. National Center for Health Statistics 1975. (Unpublished data.)

2. Health Care Financing Administration. *Long-Term Care: Background and Future Directions*, Washington, D.C.: 1981.

3. Brody, Elaine M. "Long-Term Care of the Aged: Promises and Prospects." *Health and Social Work*, 1979 *4*, pp. 30-59.

4. Granger, Carl V. "A Conceptual Model for Functional Assessment," in Carl V. Granger and Glenn E. Gresham (Eds.), *Functional Assessment in Rehabilitation Medicine*, Baltimore: Williams and Wilkens, in press.

5. World Health Organization. *International Classification of Impairments, Disabilities, and Handicaps* (ICIDH), Geneva: World Health Organization, 1980.

6. Rapoport, Lydia. "Crisis Intervention as a Mode of Treatment," in R. W. Roberts & R.H. Nee (Eds.), *Theories of Social Casework*, Chicago: University of Chicago Press, 1970, p. 295.

7. Parad, Howard S. "Crisis Intervention," in R. Morris (Ed.), *Encyclopedia of Social Work*, (Vol. 1), p. 200.

8. Rapoport, Lydia. "Crisis Intervention as a Mode of Treatment," in R. W. Roberts and R. H. Nee (Eds.), *Theories of Social Casework*, Chicago: University of Chicago Press, 1970, p. 300.

9. Golan, Naomi. *Treatment in Crisis Situations*, New York: The Free Press, 1978.

10. Ibid.

    —Speigel, D. "Crisis Points in Family Life," in A. M. Freeman, R. L. Sack, & P.A Berger (Eds.). *Psychiatry for the Primary Physician*, Baltimore: Williams and Wilkins, 1979.

11. Rossen, S. Discharge Planning-Social Workers Play an Important Role, *Social Work Administration*, 1977, *3*, pp. 4-5.

12. Shulman, Lawrence, and Tuzman, Leonard. "Discharge Planning-a Social Work Perspective," *Quality Review Bulletin*, 1980, *6*, 3-8.

13. Granger, C.V., Albrecht, G. L., and Hamilton, B. B. Outcome of Comprehensive Medical Rehabilitation: Measurement by PULSES Profile and Barthel Index," *Archives of Physical Medicine and Rehabilitation*, 1979, *60*, pp. 145-154.

14. Granger, Carl V., Sherwood, C. C., & Greer, D. S. "Functional Status Measures in a Comprehensive Stroke Program, *Archives of Physical Medicine and Rehabilitation*, 1977, *58*, pp. 555-561.

15. Fortinsky, Richard H., Granger, Carl V., Seltzer, G. B. "The Use of Functional Assessment in Understanding Home Care Needs," *Medical Care*, 1981, *19*, pp. 489-497.

16. Hollis, Florence. *Casework: a Psychosocial Therapy*, New York: Random House, 1972, p. 251.

17. Cottrell, Fred. *Aging and the Aged*, Dubuque: William C. Brown, 1974.

Huyck, M.D. *Growing Older*, Englewood Cliffs: Prentice-Hall, 1974.

18. Hubbard, R.W., Santos, J. F. and Wiora, M. "A Community-based Model for Discharge Planning and Aftercare for Hospitalized Older Adults," *Journal of Gerontological Social Work*, 1978, *1*, pp. 63-68.

Part II

CONCEPTUAL ISSUES
FOR PRACTICE

Chapter 4

SERVING FAMILIES OF THE
INSTITUTIONALIZED AGED:
THE FOUR CRISES

Renee Solomon

Entry into an institution is never an easy time for either the old person or the family. It is never easy, regardless of how the decision was made or who was involved in making it. Entry into an institution is one of life's most serious and painful crises.[1] How the social worker can help to alleviate that pain through forging alliances between the institution and family members is the focus of this chapter.

Building such an alliance is no easy task. First, it presumes an ability to relinquish the myth that families abandon their elderly relatives to institutions and to replace the myth with an appreciation of the suffering which children and their parents endure prior to placement. Second, the alliance rests upon the provision of services at those times which are most stressful for families. The elaboration and specification which follow flow from a perception of a partnership in which care of the elderly is seen as a function to be shared by families and institution.

The Myth of Abandonment

The myth that old people are abandoned by their families is finally being exploded. Shanas found that more than half (53%) of older people living in the community saw a child on that day or the day prior to the interview; approximately three-quarters (77%) had within a week.[2] Dobrof, in her study of the institutionalized aged, found that 50% were visited by relatives at least once a week; 65% twice a month, and 85% at least once a month. In addition, most talked regularly to their children by phone.[3] The nature and extent of task performance by family members is being documented in numerous studies.[4] These show that regardless of

83

age, income level or ethnic and racial background, family members minister to the emotional, social, financial, and physical needs of their elderly relatives. The accumulated evidence documents the strength of intergenerational ties, the continuity of responsible filial behavior, the frequent contacts between generations. The evidence points to the centrality of families rather than professionals in the provision of health and social services, the strenuous family efforts to avoid institutional placement of the old, and the central role played by families in caring for the noninstitutionalized impaired elderly.[5]

That most children "do the right thing" for their parents is the resounding theme of these studies. Equally important is that children are doing the right thing for many more years than ever before because their parents are living longer than have preceding generations. The demography reveals that more than a million people (mostly women) are over 85 years of age, that the oldest part of the aging population is growing the fastest, that in fact, the rate of increase of those 75 and over has escalated to three times that of people who are 65-74 years old. The average age upon entry into an institution is 83.

Statistics can belie the human dimensions of the situation which perhaps can be best understood by examining the situation of middle-aged children in an age where the four generation family is commonplace, and the five generation family no longer an anomaly.

This is the first generation in history in which numbers of people in their 40s, 50s and 60s are at one and the same time children, spouses, parents, grandparents. Dobrof refers to this position as the "intergenerational crunch" in which middle-aged children, many of them grandparents themselves, have relatives in their eighties and nineties for whom they are responsible. Some, widowed or divorced, are struggling to make a new life as a single person. Many have adult chidren who still call upon them for help. They have grandchildren for whom they babysit, or whose summer camp fees they pay, or whom they are helping to send through college. Many women have only recently returned to the work force. Indeed the modal category of working women is middle-aged married woman, a pattern which reverses the earlier one in which young and single women used to predominate the work force.[6]

Not even the most devoted children can render long-term care to their aged parents without feelings of obligation, resentment and guilt. Nor can their parents, while they know their children love and care for them, feel that they do enough. They are not free of feelings of being pushed aside, of bitterness that the children for whom they sacrificed so much cannot find time to do more for them. Old people despair that the last years should be characterized by loss of autonomy and options. The despair is often masked and expressed in behavior which their children find most painful and difficult to understand: excessive demands, preoccupation with self and apparent indifference to others, stubbornness, constant complaints and withdrawal from opportunities to be with others.[7]

Middle-aged children are experiencing their own life crises at the same time they experience the crises of their parents' lives. Too much emphasis has been placed on the quality of guilt in the feelings of middle-aged children toward their aged parents. The relationship between the 50- or 60-year-old child and her 86-year-old mother, like all other important human relationships, is a mixture of love and hate, of responsibility and resentment, of sorrow and joy, of closeness and distance.

To grow old, to face the infirmities of old age, to know that time is short, are part of the inescapable tragedy of life. It is equally tragic to watch a once strong, independent parent become old and frail and sometimes frightened and desperate, and to know that your ability to help is limited. In order for children to master the conflicts of competing claims, and for their parents to fight for integrity and against despair, the sacrifices of both parents and children must be appreciated when the move from the community to the institution is undertaken.[8]

Institutionalization

Four events can be identified as critical in the lives of the institutionalized elderly and their families. These are: (1) the decision to enter the institution, (2) entry into the institution, and (3) the move to a more intensive level of care.[9] A 4th and final crisis occurs when the old person dies. Each of these events poses a new set of developmental tasks for the old person and family, and can create or exacerbate tensions within the family unit. Institutional services which are developed to relieve the stress, and enable families to resolve these particular crises, are the means by which an alliance between the institution and the family can be forged.

Until just a few years ago there was almost complete acceptance of Shanas and Blenkners' conclusion that "no matter what the extenuating circumstances, the older person who has children interprets the move to the institution as rejection by his children."[10] Dobrof in her more recent work on the institutionalized elderly and their families reached a somewhat different conclusion. While many older people interpreted the move in this way, she found many others who themselves initiated the move, some doing so against their children's wishes. These were people who did not sanction multigeneration families living under one roof (the child's), and who could no longer maintain their own domiciles. Most people chose the institution because of declining health status, others because they tired of the forced isolation imposed by increasing frailty and danger in the streets, still others because they could no longer tolerate "being a burden" to their relatives. In examining the generalization of rejection, Dobrof makes the important distinction between those for whom this is a correct interpretation, and those for whom the decision for institutionalization reflects the family's attempt to secure the best possible care and living situation for an aged parent.[11]

The feeling of rejection however must not be minimized, and indeed even for those who choose to come, entry may feel initially like rejection. Feelings of rejection diminish when real ties are maintained with the family, when the older person sees *in fact* that she is not abandoned.[12]

The Decision to Enter

The circumstances which bring people to institutions differ markedly. Some choose to come; others have the decision made for them; some people come willingly, but see it as a temporary move. All people (and the majority of them are women), are in poor health, some with physical frailties and others with emotional or intellectual impairments. Some are able to manage by themselves, others need personal assistance and nursing care. Some have time to consider alternatives prior to entry, others find themselves transferred without warning from another institution such as an acute care hospital or mental institution. People with families tend to enter at a later age than do those without family supports. Although only 5% of people over age 65 are in institutions, one of every eight people over 80 lives in one. They are three times more likely to be single and two times more likely to be widowed than are those people who live in the community.[13]

While these different circumstances do affect the kind of help people need when they are deciding about institutionalization, the formulation of universal life tasks associated with this stressful event may be helpful in conceptualizing service needs. It is proposed that mastery of this event, the decision to enter the institution, is dependent upon the older person's ability to mobilize his/her aggressive feelings and to remain active rather than passive at this time. The decision to enter can trigger feelings of loss, which without intervention often results in depression with concomitants of helplessness and hopelessness. This can happen so easily because the decision to enter is an acknowledgment to self and others of diminished capacity to care for oneself. Whether one has chosen to enter, or has had the decision made for him/her, the older person perhaps for the first time is identified as old, sick, and frail. Social work intervention which supports or stimulates aggressive mobilization of psychological resources is needed to counteract the propensity for withdrawal.

Family members also need help. In some families the decision to enter is seen as, and is, long overdue. The primary caregiver, usually, but not in all cases, the eldest daughter, has spent agonizing years torn between her own needs, the needs of her nuclear family, and those of her parent. Some of these families are near the breaking point. In some other families, where the division of labor in caring for the parent has been seen as unfair, siblings barely speak with one another. Therefore, despite awareness of their parents distress and withdrawal, children can tend not to communicate openly about the situation. The sense is that the difficult decision about institutionalization has been made, and the newly achieved homeostasis may be upset by further discussion.

The active mediating efforts of the social worker are needed for effective family functioning. First, interventions must be directed towards connecting the family with the institution. When these efforts are underway, focus can then be placed upon resolving the interpersonal obstacles in the family unit.

Families who in this stage have access to the advice of experts including doctors and social workers have the best chance of successful placement. Selection of the proper facility is a major concern. The notion of environmental continuity[14] is helpful here. Adjustment is easier to institutional environments which are more harmonious or congruent with previous modes of functioning. Lieberman suggests that this makes a marked difference for intact persons, while it does not matter much to the more debilitated older person for whom any move increases deterioration. Staff members' demonstration of warmth and interpersonal concern were seen as key factors in environmental continuity. Additional considerations include the facility's proximity to family and friends (which encourages visiting), cultural and ethnic continuity, and of course decent medical care.

It is practice wisdom to say that preparation for life transitions such as marriage, parenthood, and retirement eases those transitions. However there have been few attempts to measure the face validity of this assertion. Stotsky who attempted such a study concluded that elderly people who were prepared for a move to an institution achieved more favorable outcomes than did those who entered peremptorily.[15]

Preparation for entry needs to be active and to go beyond imparting information. A sound appraisal of the institution by the family which includes positives and negatives is healthy, avoiding thinking about it increases helplessness. Visits to, and short stays in the facility prior to entry, are optimal. Participation of family members in some of the information sharing and visits is essential.

The expression of hurt and angry feelings must precede entry, such expression is the primary step in increasing aggression, in achieving the desired reinvolvement of the old person. Family sessions in which the social worker mediates the communication between all family members, allowing them to hear each other's pain and sorrow and their need for each other, should follow individual sessions with the parent and with the children and grandchildren. The old person and her family need to be seen as a unit, and this unit is the client. It is difficult sometimes not to see the older person as victim, the family as enemy, and social service staff as saviours. Such a rescue fantasy serves only as an impediment to service. Instead, with the entire family as the unit of attention, focus must be placed on understanding the family's feelings about placement, on easing guilt *if it is there*, on lending a vision of help, that as partners, family and institution will do what must be done to ease the pain.

Work with relatives in the stage takes two foci. First, the worker needs to understand their struggles and their position in the life cycle. What stresses other than those with elderly parents are being experienced? What has been the nature of relationship within the entire family unit? What is the family's division of labor? Who is responsible for instrumental task performance? For affective support? Who makes the decisions? What strains has care of the old person created amongst siblings? Attention here needs to be paid to the family as both a social and psychological system.

The second focus for work concerns the help we give adult children to carry on or to assume their responsibilities to parents. We are talking here of Blenkner's concept of filial maturity which marks that phase of life in which the adult child acquires the capacity to be depended on by the parent and to make his/her own transition to old age.[16] Filial maturity implies an acceptance of one's parents as they are, a recognition of their positive and negative characteristics, an acceptance of one's own positive and negative feelings towards them. Ultimately, filial maturity implies that one can no longer expect nor blame parents for whatever they have not been able to give; this resolution of anger and guilt enables adult children to enter into adult relationships with their parents. In this separateness, adult children can accept what can and cannot be done for parents, while they assume the necessary responsibilities based on kinships status. Achievement of filial maturity is enormously difficult; it is a developmental task with which the social worker can help.

The development of group services for people awaiting admission is also beneficial to familes. Group participation affords opportunities not only for information sharing, it permits people who are struggling with similar issues to help each other in their struggles. The comfort received from peers as part of the mutual aid process cannot be replicated by professionals or friends or children. Group participation also allows for the development of new friendships or acquaintanceships which can ease the pain of entry into the institution.

None of the above may be possible for families of the person who is peremptorily transferred from the acute care hospital to the long-term care facility. While the number of people in this category varies with location (it was as high as 45% in the Chicago study done by Tobin & Lieberman), we do know that the foreshortened waiting period for the intact person increases the incidence of depression and other negative effects. While it is no easy task to accomplish, it is suggested that the transfer with no prior notice need not occur. In cases where utilization review is used as basis for discharge, the hospital social worker must be creative in individualizing the client by bending the rules so that discharge is delayed.[17] The social worker in the long-term care facility needs to delay admission, again either by obtaining sanction for it, or if that is not possible, by bending rules, so that time is gained for a visit to the person in the hospital during which time a quick but personal orientation to the facility can be made. Empathy for the older person's lack of choice needs to be communicated at this time. The family too needs to be contacted and urged to visit the institution immediately prior to their relative's admission.

Admission Into the Institution

All of the mixed feelings which characterize close human relationships may surface upon entry into the institution. This is a time of crisis as the old person and her family face the reality of her declining health status. This is a time of crisis—in which everyone is aware that it is the last move which the older person will make.

The developmental task which accompanies the crisis of admission is that of maintaining close family ties while feeling angry, hurt, afraid of rejection and abandonment, and most of all, feeling deeply sorrowful. Parents and their children all are grieving for the passing of an era. And they do this while simultaneously confronting their own mortality. Is it any wonder that when faced with these two issues, which may feel life-threatening to some, that the impulse can be one of flight? Depending upon the strength of family relationships, the extent of open communication, and patterns of coping with crisis, families may react to this current crisis by coming together or pulling apart. For the old person entering the institution, fears of abandonment become reality when children are not helped to stay close even in the face of their own desire to withdraw. For their children, a little help in continuing to "do the right thing" helps to relieve the hurt, or perhaps shame or guilt for being angry with a now "helpless" parent.

Institutional procedures which require family members to stay close during the first few weeks after admission are helpful to families. Such procedures send implicit messages that long-term care is a shared function, that family involvement is essential to institutional adjustment, that family members are welcome in their parents' home. Having at least one family member spend the entire first day at the Home is suggested, as are daily visits by as many family members as possible for the first two weeks. These behaviors visibly demonstrate the continuity of commitment; they may serve to alleviate the children's guilt and their parents' fears of abandonment.

Such an extensive family presence may however pose problems for the institution. Relatives can "get underfoot," "raise questions," "take time" which busy staff members cannot spare. Notwithstanding this reality, client need must supersede system maintenance needs. Many service systems intensify the misery they are intended to mitigate. Many nursing homes institutionalize despair; hospitals are not fit places to be sick in, etc. Institutions, including those for the elderly, seem to move inevitably and ineluctably towards greater concern with their own maintenance than with their intended purpose. All the disappointments and inadequacies to which all service systems are heir to are presided over by decent professional people (like our readers and ourselves), not by easy-to-despise villains. It is the unwitting bad done by the "good" people that really complicates things for the elderly, not the intended evil of the "bad" people.[18]

Institutional policies and procedures which encourage the maintenance of family ties are operationalized in many ways—by open visiting hours, by providing facilities like coffee shops and lounges where families can spend time with one another, by encouraging families to bring special food treats, by minimizing obstacles for visits to homes of relatives and so forth. Staff members with the best will in the world may not be sensitive to institutional obstacles to maintenance of family relationships. Social workers need to make certain that channels of communication between institution staff and families remain open. We need to understand how institutional systems work so that informed attention can be paid to influencing them so that they work for clients.

Maintaining close contact during the admission period helps mitigate feelings of abandonment. Feelings of rejection which differ from abandonment, may be lessened when control and autonomy remain with the older person. Wherever possible decisions about financial matters, personal belongings, and participation in activities should be made by the old person. Such "simple" matters as the hanging up of clothes, display of family pictures etc., can become conflictual areas as children seek to "do for their parents," while most parents although physically unable to perform these tasks, do know how they want them done. Family members need help in learning to ask for and follow the directions of their elderly relatives. Rooms should be arranged (even though shared), according to the residents' desires; the new resident should be allowed to make the initial approach to the roommate and to others on the floor. Institutional life, ipso facto decreases decision-making opportunities— what to eat, with whom to eat, when to eat etc. Within these parameters, we want to preserve people's ability to make the small decisions, to maintain whatever degree of control is possible over their lives. Autonomy is dignity; its absence grades and confirms one's disadvantaged status.

A range of counselling services which begin on the day of admission need to be put in place. Units of attention include younger family members, the old person, the old person and her family. In addition, family groups for families of all new residents and groups for new residents are essential to helping families deal with their feelings, and to perform the tasks which attend institutionalization.

The admission crisis while it may look different has some fairly universal components. Family members tend to feel guilt; the old person tends to feel rejected and enraged. These latter feelings need to be contained for the fear of abandonment is also present. Therefore they get covered over with statements like "I don't want to be a burden." "Don't come so much. I know you're busy," "It's my choice to live here, and I'll manage." Covering, which is a form of coping can be highly dysfunctional: (1) it serves to bottle up feelings which can in turn lead to depression, (2) it can increase children's guilt feelings which can lead to withdrawal, and (3) it diverts precious energy needed to cope with the demands of the new living situation.

Family members must be helped to express and accept resentment and anger without being overwhelmed by guilt. "They must be helped to tolerate abuse or to withdraw gracefully."[19] The worker in individual family and group counselling sessions should focus on the expression of feelings, positive and negative, should validate the enormity of the adjustment issues, and should support all efforts to maintain the family unit. Efforts must be directed to understanding the familial coping patterns and most particularly the strengths of the family unit and this unique old person. Once again, the social worker as mediator is there to connect family members with each other, and to connect the family to needed institutional resources. The worker in new residents groups needs to sanction "complaining" and encourage participation in group services which have a change focus. Such participation augments power and control issues discussed earlier.

In concluding this section it is important to make the explicit implicit, and to note that resolution of the admission crisis is dependent upon three interrelated sets of variables. First there are the environmental support systems which the institution brings to bear, second there is the family's ability to use these services, and third, we have the unique qualities of the person entering the institution.

The Move to a More Intensive Level of Care

Although entry into the long-term care facility made all family members encounter their own mortality, life after admission served to dilute fears of imminent death. Efforts have been directed to the quality of life, and adjustments have been made. For some families, as Simos points out, relationships improved as children no longer panicked with each phone call, knowing that their parents were safe. Some children for the first time, had the opportunity to see parents make a new and good life and marveled at the strength their parents possessed. In other families, relationships were ruptured and the children have withdrawn emotionally, or physically or both. In some families where affective ties have lessened, children become important in different ways—they come to be seen as symbols of success and as carrying on the family tradition and values.[20]

The need for a more intensive level of care, which may come gradually or quite suddenly, once again brings the family face-to-face with issues of death and dying. At this stage the issue is more real and needs to be faced, even though death itself may not be imminent.

The developmental task for the elderly with increased health debilitation is that of resolving the issue of integrity versus despair. Children and their parents have this opportunity to finish their unfinished business, to find resolution of the pulls and tensions, to come to terms with life as it was. The resolution of integrity versus despair in the Ericksonian sense is the "acceptance of one's one and only life cycle as something that had to be, and that by necessity, permitted of no substitution."[21] Families need to be educated to this major task of aging. They need to understand that if their parents are to escape despair, they and their parents must be able to accept that what was, was—that now, there is the reality that what was, cannot be altered.

Achievement of integrity, and the freedom from despair is the elderly parents' task. It requires that the old person give up the luxury which is permissible earlier—the luxury of "it would have been different if we weren't so poor," or "it would have been different if I hadn't driven him away" or "it would have been different if we had not married and had kids when we were so young." This luxury is permitted us when we were younger, according to Erickson, for then there is still time to start another life; to try out alternative roads to integrity.

The despair experienced by the elder whose frailty is palpable is often marked with constant complaints about poor treatment, and with self absorption. As with earlier crises, this one can also provoke flight in family members who themselves are distraught and impotent in the face of increased mental and/or physical infirmity. There is the added problem of not knowing what to talk about when visiting. The elder is often focussed only upon self, his/her world is limited to his/her room or he/she may not be as intact mentally as before. As Jack Weinberg asked "What do you say to mother when you have nothing to say."[22] Help to families in coping with this crisis can take the form of educational workshops on the therapeutic function of reminiscence.

Reminiscence, the act of recalling and narrating past experiences is an important vehicle for resolving the issue of integrity versus despair. Family members can be taught to appreciate its significance and to engage in the act of reminiscence with elderly relatives.[23] Recalling painful struggles, the joyous times, the manifold relationships, also helps to rekindle feelings of mastery and power, feelings which are all too frequently absent from the aged person's current existence. Reminiscence is a vehicle whereby the wholeness of one's life, the integrity of one's self is preserved. To remember coming to America alone at age 17 to avoid the draft in Czarist Russia, the ensuing struggles to survive, to marry and to raise a family; to remember trade union struggles or the building of a business; to remember mothering a family, struggling to make ends meet; to remember the accolades of an achievement, is at least during the moments of remembering, to once again count as a contributing human being.

Participation in and encouragement of family reminiscing can bring families closer together. The elderly relative is given the opportunity to be valued in her entirety with strengths as well as weaknesses and dependencies. Younger people are given the chance to learn from the struggles of the past and to preserve those struggles. And for the family, reminiscence becomes the family legacy; it can ensure family continuity; it is the preservation of the past which ensures the future.

Families may also need help at this time in facing issues of death and dying, and, if the illness is terminal, in saying good-bye to their parents. The literature on death/dying makes the compelling point that for most old people, death is feared far less than is abandonment. Families need help to visit and when this becomes too painful, they need sanction to come less frequently. Social workers need to assume the role of surrogate families, easing burdens for those who can no longer carry them, while appreciating the impulses of those who come beyond the time, when in our professional judgment, it is no longer necessary to do so. Easy access to workers is essential at this time.

Dying in the Institution

Too often the death of the resident signifies the end of service to families. But families survive the death of parents and they need our help in working through their loss and in achieving a new equilibrium. By virtue of the close ties which have been maintained between families and institutions in the care of the elderly, the abrupt severing of relationships on the day of death or the funeral is experienced by families as uncaring, as bureaucratic, as abandonment.

Although an old person's death is "in its season," unlike the death of a younger person, most families are not prepared for the death, or for their own possibly strong reactions to it. The death of one's remaining parent can leave one feeling like an orphan (and literally one is), at the age of 50 or even 60 or 70. The mantle of head of family has been passed on; new role relationships need to be established. The social worker needs to be available to help families with their grief work, understanding that it will be different for each family. Grieving will be affected by factors such as centrality to the unit of the person who has died, the nature of death, the length of illness, the openness of communication within the family unit.

In death, the partnership of family and institution is evidenced also by the ways in which the death is marked in the institution. When staff attend funerals and are available to help the bereaved, when attention to death is paid in the institution by announcements, by special services, by making provision for other residents to attend the funeral, then the value of their relative's life is affirmed to the family.

Conclusion

To say that all family relationships are different, that each reflects a history, that all can change over time given the presence or absence of needed resources, is to risk concluding with the obvious. Still, anyone who studies aging, the elderly, or family relationships of the elderly concludes that no single conclusion can be deduced from them or it.

We have nevertheless attempted to delineate the major crises which accompany institutionalization and to specify the array of services which can help families cope with these crises. The departure point for this chapter has been that of a partnership between the institution and families in caring for the elderly. Such a partnership insures that the resident retains family and community ties, and insures accountability of family and institution each to the other. As Dobrof observed, institutions which welcome families as partners, which take into account the psychological tensions in family relationships, and yet still encourage families to do what they can and what they believe they should, are articulating ethical imperatives of responsibility which govern intergenerational relationships. "And this is a payoff, the value of which can neither be measured with precision, nor underestimated."[24]

REFERENCES

1. Dobrof, Rose & Litwak, Eugene. *Maintenance of Family Ties of Long Term Care Patients: Theory & Guide to Practice*, (Rockville Md: National Institute of Mental Health, Department of Health, Education & Welfare), 1977.

2. Shanas, Ethel. "Social Myth as Hypothesis," *The Gerontologist, 19,* 1979, p.p. 3-9.

3. Dobrof, Rose. "The Care of the Aged: A Shared Function," Unpublished Doctoral Dissertation, Columbia University School of Social Work, 1976.

4. See for example, Marjorie Cantor. "Caring for the Frail Elderly: Impact on Family, Friends and Neighbors." Mattesich, Paul and Mederer, Helen, 1980. "Family Interaction and Perception of Need Among the Elderly and Their Children."; Mellor, Joanna and Getzel, George, 1980. "Stress and Service Needs of Those Who Care for the Aged." Papers presented at the Thirty-Third Annual Scientific Meeting, Gerontological Society, San Diego, California, 1980.

5. Brody, Elaine L. "Women in the Middle" and "Family Help to Older People," *Gerontologist 21,* 1981, p.p. 471-480.

6. Bengston, V. & Deterre, E. "Aging & Family Relations" *Marriage & Family Review 3,* 1980, p.p. 51-76.

7. Solomon, Renee. "Aging Individuals in L.T.C. Need Choice & Autonomy," *Generations 5,* 1979, p.p. 32-34.

8. Studies of the nature & extent of stress experienced by children who perform tasks for elderly parents over time are currently being undertaken. See for example, Amy Horowitz, 1982, "Adult Children as Caregivers to Elderly Parents: Correlates & Consequences," Unpublished Doctoral Dissertation, Columbia University School of Social Work.

9. Tobin, Sheldon, & Lieberman, Martin. *Last Home for the Aged.* San Francisco: Jossey Bass, 1976.

10. Blenkner, Margaret. "Social Work and Family Relationships in Later Life with Some Thoughts on Filial Maturity." In: E. Shanas, and G. Streib, Eds. *Social Structure and the Family: Generational Relations.* Englewood Cliffs, N.J.: Prentice-Hall, 1965. p.p. 46-62.

11. Dobrof, & Litwak, *op.cit.*

12. Brody. *Op.cit.*

13. Shanas. *Op.cit.*

14. Tobin, & Lieberman, *op.cit.*

15. Stotsky, B.A. "Social & Clinical Issues in Geriatric Psychiatry" *American Journal of Psychiatry 129,* 1972, p.p. 117-126.

16. Blenkner. *Op.cit.*

17. Miller. Irving, Presentation *Alumni Conference,* Columbia University School of Social Work, 1973.

18. Miller, Irving, & Solomon, R. "The Development of Group Services for the Elderly" in Carel Germain Ed. *Social Work Practice: People & Environments.* Columbia University Press, 1979.

19. Tobin, & Lieberman. *Op.cit.*

20. Simos, Bertha. "Adult Children and their Aging Parents" *Social Work 18,* May 1973. p.p. 78-85.

21. Erikson, Erik. *Childhood & Society,* New York: W.W. Norton, 1963.

22. Weinberg, Jack. "What Do I Say to My Mother When I Have Nothing to Say" in Marie Blank & S. Steury Eds. *Readings in Psychotherapy with Older People.* Rockville, Md.: National Institute of Mental Health, Department of Health, Education & Welfare, 1977.

23. Miller, & Solomon, *op.cit.*

24. Dobrof, 1977. *Op.cit.*

Chapter 5

ETHICAL DILEMMAS IN LONG-TERM CARE

Harry R. Moody

Ethical dilemmas are unavoidable in the practice of social work today. Social work practice in long-term care settings presents many of the ethical problems encountered by social workers elsewhere, as well as some special problems associated with old age or with the management of institutionalized dependent groups of people.

The substantive issues of social work ethics in general can be divided into several broad patterns, following Reamer and Abramson.[1]

1. *Services to Individuals, Families and Groups.* Ethical issues here concern such problems as when to maintain absolute confidentiality and privacy; the obligation of truth telling and the prohibition never to lie; the conflict between paternalism (doing what's best for the client) versus self-determination; adherence to laws, policies, and regulations (obeying orders); the dilemma of divided professional loyalties (e.g., the professional codes versus employers, colleagues, etc.); and the problem of allocating limited resources among clients or groups of clients.

2. *Social Welfare Policy and Programs.* When social workers act at levels beyond the individual client, they unavoidably encounter a series of ethical issues such as: the status of welfare rights (what are people entitled to?); the proper role and limits of government power; the dilemmas of distributive justice; and the relation between social injustice and the priorities of the social work profession.

3. *Dilemmas Among Professional Colleagues.* Social workers in long-term care settings have as colleagues, both other social workers and members of different professional groups (nurses, doctors, physical therapists, etc.). Ethical problems here include: whistle-blowing (revealing patterns of wrong-doing); the use of deception; the status of privileged

---

[1]See Reamer and Abramson, *Teaching of Social Work Ethics*, for a more extensive discussion of these substantive issues, which are drawn directly from their formulation.

communications (confidentiality with fellow-professionals); and the resolution of interdisciplinary conflicts.[2]

Finally, overriding all these issues there are recurrent questions that
are at the center of moral philosophy and moral action. For example.
what is the status of our beliefs about moral obligation? Are these obligations grounded in pure reason, in human nature, in social convention
or on some other basis? Secondly, even if we can be sure about the
foundations of our moral beliefs, what do we do when obligations or
different values begin to conflict with one another? How do we make
decisions in practice when *our own* beliefs on a matter are in conflict—
in short, when we're ambivalent about what to do? These, in brief,
are some recurrent questions that social workers will encounter, and they
serve as an appropriate background to any detailed consideration of social
work ethical dilemmas in long-term care.

Ethical dilemmas in long-term care begin with the question of whether
there should be long-term care facilities at all. There are those who
believe, on ideological or philosophical grounds, that families should
"take care of their own" (an opinion popular among conservatives), or,
alternatively, that government should provide funds for home-health care
so that no elderly person would ever have to enter a nursing home (an
opinion popular among liberals). As to the first opinion—that nursing
homes would not be necessary in conditions of genuine family responsibility—the answer is that such a view fails to take account of the enormous
hidden costs, trade-offs, and value dilemmas involved in family caregiving: for example, sacrifice of the well-being of adult children, of
elderly spouses, of grandchildren, and so on. Then too there are the large
numbers of elderly without any family supports to rely on. A rigorous
policy *against* support of nursing homes involves very serious ethical
problems, but they cannot be dealt with here. What is clear enough is
that, over a generation or more, public policy in the U.S. has decided
in favor of nursing homes as care-giving institutions for the frail and
impaired elderly. Given that state of affairs, a range of ethical dilemmas
will arise.

There are other critics who are unhappy with nursing homes because
those facilities are "total institutions" in the sense defined by sociologist
Erving Goffman or historian David Rothman. Like mental hospitals,
nursing homes easily become instruments of social control and like other
total institutions, nursing homes routinely fail to safeguard basic rights of
patients. In this view, it is not episodic scandals of fraud or abuse but the
very institutions themselves that are an indictment of our society's re-

sponse to the elderly. Instead of inhumane institutional care, these critics call for a vast expansion of publicly supported home-health care to enable the elderly to live in their own homes (the "least restricted environment") as long as possible.

Like the conservative appeal to family responsibility, the liberal critique also appeals to cherished moral values—autonomy, self-determination, individual rights. And, as with the appeal to family responsibility, the call for home-health care overlooks enormous costs, trade-offs, and value dilemmas associated with public policy favoring de-institutionalization. We will return to this issue at the end of this discussion when, I believe, it will become apparent that most of the ethical issues in long-term care facilities reappear when care is shifted to the home.

A Taxonomy of Ethical Issues

Long-term care for the elderly—both in nursing homes and in home-health care settings—presents a range of ethical dilemmas that professionals will not fail to confront in practice.

- Is it right to systematically mislabel clients in order to help them qualify for eligibility for services provided on the basis of "need"? For which clients and under which circumstances?
- Does one have an obligation to report cases of abuse, neglect, or mistreatment of patients in nursing homes? To inform higher officials or go to the press with the information?
- Is it proper to restrict admission to a given nursing home according to a patient's race or religion? According to their prior or current monetary contribution to the home?
- Is it proper for professionals to receive gifts from patients' families? From patients themselves?
- Should staff members intervene to encourage a patient to make a specific decision in favor of a treatment plan or in favor of participating or not participating in a clinical research program?

How the social worker responds to those ethical dilemmas will depend, at least in part, on whether the ethical issues are recognized and on how one has learned to think about such issues. It is too much to claim that merely recognizing, describing, or analyzing problems will lead to their resolution. Yet without some overlook "taxonomy" of the issues, we cannot hope to make much progress in dealing with them.

Thus, in thinking about ethical dilemmas in long-term care settings it is helpful to make the following distinctions:

Source of the Problem. Is the issue we confront one that originates in long-term care settings themselves, or does it arise from some other factor—advanced old age, mental frailty, chronic illness, or terminal disease?

Ethical Dilemma or Practical Problem? Is the issue we confront a genuine ethical dilemma or is it rather a problem of implementation? In other words, are we unclear about what *is* the right thing to do or simply unable to carry out a solution?

Professional Perspective. How is the ethical issue framed by our perspective of professional practice (the view of social work in contrast to nursing, medicine, etc.)? How does a professional perspective help (or hinder) the clarification of empirical and normative features of the situation?

Level of Action. What is the appropriate level of social action where ethical dilemmas appear and find resolution? Is it at the policy level, the professional practice level, or the level of individual beliefs and values?

Ethical Theory. How can ethical theories help clarify the dilemma and its range of possible resolutions? Is it a matter of basic human *rights*, of *utility*, of individual *virtue*, or of *social justice*?

Source of the Problem

Some ethical dilemmas—for example, those associated with death and dying—arise inevitably at the end of a long lifespan, regardless of institutional settings.

> An 85-year-old patient, who decides not to undergo a painful chemo-therapy regimen may or may not be making a good decision; in fact, may or may not even be judged capable of making a decision (for example, a patient with advanced chronic brain syndrome). Long-term care settings do not create this patient's problem, but, if the patient is a resident of a nursing home, then staff may be-come involved in the patient's decision-making (e.g., giving advice to the family, counselling the patient, etc.)

The case of a patient's decision to pursue or not to pursue chemotherapy already indicates a connection with a recommended medical procedure, and therefore, with a degree of institutional involvement in the decision itself. Are we justified in describing such a negative decision as an act of "suicide," or, more mildly, "voluntary euthanasia"?[3] The question itself indicates the ethical significance that labelling can have in framing the terms of our moral judgment. We are inclined to approve of a patient's right to self-determination in decisions over medical care, whereas if we describe the same mental act as a decision to commit suicide, we are likely to think that psychiatric help is called for.

> A 78-year-old patient, resident of a nursing home for three years, announces to the social worker that she no longer wants to live, that she wants the worker's help in obtaining excess doses of sleeping pills in order to end her life quietly. Should the social worker report this request to a psychiatrist or medical director? Should the social worker keep it confidential and do nothing? Should the social worker attempt to talk the resident out of her depression, provide counselling, and so on? Should the social worker help the patient carry our her express wish to end her life (e.g., obtain doses of sleeping pills)?

The instance above shows a decision initiated independently by a nursing home resident without response to medical procedures recommended by institutional staff. Nevertheless, the institutional staff—the social worker—is now involved in the decision. The social worker is caught in a dilemma: he or she cannot pretend "not to have heard" the resident's wish. But what to do about it? And how far is this an institutional matter at all?

By contrast, there are other ethical issues that are *intrinsically* institutional actions in the sense that the decisions are generated by the existence of the institutional setting itself: for example, when a nursing home makes decisions about preferential admission in accepting applicants outside the waiting list, or when staff members become aware of patterns of patient abuse and neglect. The first is an issue of *distributive justice* (allocation of scarce resources),[4] and raises questions of fairness; the second is an issue of institutional loyalty, confidentiality, and obligations to patients.[5]

What makes the problem confusing is that the same dilemma can arise from one or more of the following quite different sources:

Advanced Old Age. How much longer can a patient be expected to live even under the best of circumstances (an actuarial criterion)? Should age itself affect our ethical decision-making?

Terminal Illness. A sizable proportion of nursing home residents will die within a year or two, making nursing homes into a kind of *de facto* "hospice" setting.

Chronic Illness. With disabilities, mental competency may be unimpaired but the patient will be "incompetent" to carry out his or her intentions.

Mental Frailty. These range from mild short-term memory loss to severe senile dementia, which impairs the power of reasoned choice.

Institutional Setting. All institutional life requires fixed rules of procedure (menus, daily schedules, physical safety requirements), that limit liberty. Further pressures of conformity or intimidation may severely restrict individual freedom.

It often happens that all five of these elements are present in the same patient's situation, but they are analytically distinct and should be kept so. The presence or absence of one factor or another may be crucial. Mental impairment, for example, may justify special professional interventions (e.g., protective services, guardianship, and so on), while no such intervention is called for in cases of chronic illness which leaves informed consent intact. Failure to be clear about the *source* of a patient's problem—which calls for an empirical answer—may lead to a deeper failure in ethical analysis—since normative resolution will depend, in part, on our accuracy in describing the empirical situation. "Facts" and "values," in other words, cannot be entirely separated.

Ethical Dilemma or Practical Problem?

Problems we always have with us: as Freud remarked, "Life is a problem for everybody." But ethical dilemmas are another matter, and we need to be clear about the difference. Is the situation we face a genuine ethical dilemma—a clash between opposing ethical principles— or is it merely that we lack resources to carry out a clear solution to the problem?

Consider the case of an elderly stroke patient who cannot walk easily. Given the patient's clinical situation, it is reasonable to ask whether this patient can benefit from physical therapy (in principle, an empirical question). If the answer is "yes," but no such services are available in the particular facility where the patient lives, then we are faced with a practical problem of how to help the patient get the needed services. *But*, if the patient would not qualify for therapy under existing reimbursement criteria, then, we may be faced with an ethical question of whether or not to "stretch" our account of the patient's condition in order to help the patient qualify for physical therapy. The ethical dilemma is whether or not it is right to mislabel or misrepresent the facts in order to accomplish a morally worthwhile purpose (a dilemma of truth-telling)?

This case raises a more fundamental issue that ought to be examined regardless of whether we face a "dilemma" or merely a "problem." Why is there difficulty in putting a treatment plan into effect when needed resources are not available? Why is it that the social worker is faced with a moral dilemma of choosing either to lie or see the patient fail to get needed services? If we simply "muddle through" by pragmatically doing our best, or again, if we decide simply either to lie (or not to lie), then we keep our sights too narrowly focused on the micro-issue in front of us. Instead, we need to look at *both* ethical dilemmas and implementation problems in a larger context. These micro-issues take on meaning within a larger, pre-existing context created by Medicare reimbursement formulas, licensing of physical therapists, and the distribution of income and power among professions, facilities, patients and their families.

Professional Perspectives. Each profession represented on the staff of long-term care facilities—medicine, nursing, social work, and so on—sees the patient through a distinctive "lense" of its own assumptions, methodologies, and norms of professional action. The professional's scope of action is already rule-governed by principles of professional codes of ethics (Hippocratic Oath, NASW Code, etc.,)[6] and by informal norms enforced by colleagues. The physician's perspective tends to be dominated by technical rules (diagnosis and cure), while the nurse's perspective is dominated by bureaucratic patterns (following orders), blended with hands-on support (caring). The social worker's perspective tends to be dominated by a holistic impulse for conflict-resolution, mediation, and balancing competing interests in the situation. Each of these cognitive styles—the technical, the rule-governed, the mediating—succeeds in avoiding the controversy associated with genuine ethical dilemmas. Each professional style, in short, is not only a way or dealing with value issues but also a way of escaping from those value issues that are most perplexing. When real conflicts arise, codes of ethics generally give no clue as to how to reconcile competing principles.

Level of Action

When faced with ethical dilemmas, it is essential to *locate* the dilemma at the proper scale, as in the injunction of tracing back micro-issues to the macro-context in which they arise. Some issues can only be resolved at the *policy* level (e.g., whether to provide public funding for home health care), but, regardless of policy considerations, ethical dilemmas arise at the level of professional *practice* and of *individual value* commitments (e.g., counselling an older person about entering a nursing home and considering whether I would want to live in one myself).

> A good example of the interrelationship of the three levels appears in current discussion of family care-giving. A *policy* perspective might encourage family care-giving and keeping the frail elderly at home, justified either by an appeal to autonomy or cost-effectiveness, or both. A *practice* perspective might confront the same problem by case management to draw on informal support systems, perhaps encountering value dilemmas associated with distribution of the burden of care on different family members. Finally, an *individual* perspective might stress my own personal belief in filial responsibility and inter-generational obligations: a duty of gratitude toward my parents.

In distinguishing among these different levels of action, we can see that different ethical principles—autonomy, professional duty, gratitude, and so on—come into play at different levels of action. A principle of utility—"cost-effectiveness"—may play a role on the policy level but not on the individual level; a principle of gratitude or individual equity may appear at the individual level but not at the policy level. It is a clear failure of ethical thinking for a social worker to confuse normative propositions that are valid at one level but not at another.

> Nursing home admissions staff often encounter a situation in which an elderly person has consulted with an attorney and arranged to transfer large financial assets—stocks and bonds, for example— in order to lower their personal assets to a point where the person can qualify for Medicaid to pay for nursing home care. An individual admissions staff member may well be morally outraged that such "unfairness" can occur: that is, the elderly applicant isn't "really" poor at all but qualifies because of a legal loophole in the

Medicaid law. Yet is seems an improper use of one's professional position to pass judgement on how an individual makes use of perfectly legal entitlements. From a professional practice standpoint, it would be wrong to discourage or oppose admission of the individual who has "unfairly" taken advantage of the Medicaid entitlement by transfering assets.

The transfer of assets example above clearly shows how confusing levels—policy versus professional versus individual—can lead to inappropriate actions. To say this is not to deny that the value dilemma involved here is real and may be painful for an admissions staff member.

Ethical Theories

What do we do when confronted with a genuine ethical dilemma—say, in truth-telling, or in ending a person's life, or in allocating scarce resources? Historically, the philosophical discipline of ethics has sought to clarify these questions by an analysis of practical reasoning applied to ethical dilemmas. Philosophical ethics, in short, is not a collection of pious goals that we all agree upon but instead a *procedure* for dealing with disputes arising when people disagree about what is the right thing to do. Some ethical theories—notably, skepticism, relativism, and nihilism—have maintained that there is no answer corresponding to the question of what is "the right thing to do." But historically, philosophers have largely rejected the views of skepticism, relativism, and nihilism and have acknowledged that *good reasons* play a central role in resolving ethical disputes. More to the point, when social workers or others disagree among themselves about what is "the right thing to do" in ethical dilemmas of long-term care, the existence of the argument itself demonstrates an appeal to "good reason" in support of a proposed course of action. Here it is helpful to distinguish several different kinds of reasons or ethical theories that can be advanced.

1. *Human Rights*. Alongside professional codes of ethics (e.g., NASW code of Ethics), there exist documents such as the "Nursing Home Patient's Bill of Rights." A patient's *rights* evidently are correlative to certain *duties* owed either by institutions or professionals or both. For example, a patient in a long-term care facility may be said to have a "right to die" (that is, a right not to be forced to have their life prolonged against their will). A similar case is made for the "right to be told the truth" (for informed consent), "the right to self-determination"

(in working out a treatment plan), a "right to fair treatment in the facility" and so on. All these rights on the part of the patient would generate *prima facie* duties on the part of the social worker: e.g., the duty to tell the truth, the duty to support the patient's wish not to be kept alive, and so on.

An ethical theory of basic human rights, along with prima facie duties has obvious appeal. But serious problems immediately arise. Even if we can all agree on a list of "basic rights" belonging to patients in a long-term care setting, how would those rights be enforced? Second, what do we do when rights themselves conflict with one another or with the rights of other persons? How do we decide which rights have priority and what would constitute a good reason for giving up one right in favor of another?

The theory of basic human rights can be justified by more global principles, such as a Judeo-Christian concept of human dignity, the doctrine of natural rights, or a Kantian version of the Golden Rule (Categorical Imperative). Perhaps more global principles might indicate good reasons for establishing priorities among competing rights, but unless legal machinery exists for enforcing such ethical rights, then rights, in practice, may have little meaning.

2. *Utility.* Social workers are readily attracted by versions of the theory of Utilitarianism: the ethical doctrine that customs, practices, and laws are to be judged by whether they produce a maximum benefit in human welfare for the greatest number of people, where "each person is to count for one, no person for more than one." Utilitarianism fits in well with progressive ideologies of social welfare, democracy, and egalitarianism. But utilitarianism also fits in well with the contemporary goal of "rational management" in health and human services, and this point is the basis for its appeal to administrators. Principles such as an "appropriate placement" (on a continuum of care) can be justified but so can "cost-effectiveness" as a reason for withdrawing scarce services. Justification for social work intervention through the utilitarian goal of maximizing welfare (or happiness or "life satisfaction") can be used by both reformers and defenders of the status quo.

One major problem with utilitarianism in the field of aging is that, applied consistently, it seems to hold out little reason for investing any resources in care of the very old or the very sick. If our criterion is "the greatest good for the greatest number" (whatever that may mean), then limited resources dictate a "triage" strategy: give scarce health care resources only to those who can benefit from the resources. No expensive coronary bypass operations for eighty-year-old patients. In fact, some

welfare states (e.g., Sweden and Great Britain) already have rules pro-
hibiting expensive surgical procedures for persons over a fixed age.
A similar utilitarian logic was once used in the U.S. to deny false teeth
to the elderly: why bother fitting the teeth when old people wouldn't
have many years to make use of them? Utilitarianism, when advocated
on a rigorous and consistent basis, seems to do violence to some of our
most fundamental ethical ideals of justice, fair-treatment, truth-telling,
and so on. At least, those ethical ideals can be supported only as long as
they continue to generate maximum social benefit. Judged on such a
harsh criterion, the elderly in long-term care settings might fare poorly
indeed.

3. *Virtue*. Ethical theories of rights and utility seek good reasons that
would justify a system of rules by which we could order the activities of
institutions and individuals. But "rules" and "principles" are not the only
ingredients of ethical action. For ethical action to arise in the first place
requires certain capacities or dispositions on the part of an agent: an
individual who thinks or deliberates about different courses of action.
The first such disposition—or virtue—is the capacity to recognize ethical
issues in the first place. The sense of individual ethical responsibility,
the distinction between a practical problem, and an ethical dilemma, the
capacity to envisage alternative principles, to see "good reasons" for opposing courses of action: all of these are *virtues* which practical reasoning
demands. Similarly, even if we are capable of thinking correctly about
what is "the right thing to do" we must also be capable of carrying out
our decision. Hence, virtues of reliability, truthfulness, and courage become essential.

> The virtue of courage becomes especially significant in the case
> where a social worker is cognizant of improper actions—say, abuse
> of patients—on the part of co-workers, or where a pattern of im-
> proper action—say, receiving bribes or "gifts"—becomes endemic
> within a given nursing home. In such a case, the social worker
> may conclude what must be done yet be unable to carry out the
> decision. "Whistle-blowing" requires courage that is balanced by
> good judgment, and both of these are imperative virtues.

Another dimension of virtue is apparent when we reflect on what
an ethical dilemma actually means. By definition, when a social worker
is faced with a genuine moral dilemma, *there is no automatic rule* for
giving preference to one moral principle (e.g., human rights) over another

(e.g., utility). Ethical dilemmas, in short, are "hard cases" (in the lawyers' jargon), and in a well-known aphorism of law, "hard cases make bad law." But in chronic and terminal illness, in conditions of fluctuating mental competency, in short, in the circumstances of long-term care, the social worker will repeatedly be faced with such hard cases. The solution is *not* to opt for a single-minded principle for rule-governed ethical decision-making, but to accept that, in many instances, principles and rules will contradict one another. The resolution can only be based on a judgment of what the "equity" of the situation demands, and this calls for skilled appraisal based on practical judgment.

> It will occasionally happen that persons in a long-term care facility express different views at different times concerning a clinical treatment plan. For example, when a resident refuses to take prescribed medication. Should the social worker pass on this information to the medical staff or keep the information secret? Should the social worker help "persuade" the person to "take their medicine" or act as a "patient advocate," perhaps enlisting the family as allies? A pure principle of informed consent (right to refuse treatment) might indicate one course of action, while a pure utilitarian approach could indicate that the patient's own welfare is best served by persuasion. In an actual case, the "equity" of the situation will be unclear. Ultimately, the social worker must decide what his or her ethical stance will be. But a case-by-case approach requires a well-developed virtue of good judgment.

4. *Social Justice.* We have seen that not all ethical problems can be reduced to issues of rights or justice. There will always be an irreducible scope for discretion, for charity, for courage: in short, for the virtues. Yet to state the problem of ethics this way leaves open a broader question. What kind of society, what conditions of social justice, will promote *both* the fair allocation of scarce resources (a matter of justice), *and* the flourishing of individual personality (a matter of virtue)? Justice, in this sense, is the first and primary virtue of organized human society.

The concept of social justice applied to long-term care presents many difficulties. Proponents of an egalitarian theory of justice—such as John Rawls—are likely to see health care as a "basic good" that should be made widely available.[7] In keeping with the priority of liberty, long-term care for the elderly should give preference to home-health care or other settings which are less restrictive than total institutions. More conservatively inclined thinkers—such as Robert Nozick—are inclined to leave all such decisions up to individuals and their families, who can provide the care themselves or purchase it in the free market. Between these views, and alongside them, will be many other social policy perspectives based on fundamental concepts of what a just society might look like.

For the practitioner—say, the social worker employed in a long-term care facility—these opposing concepts of social justice will present themselves in a more practical way. The laws, regulations, and conditions of work in the field of long-term care will display a series of contradictions between intent of legislation and method of implementation; among the different levels of policy, practice, and individual judgment; and even between basic ethical principles themselves.

The social worker must be able to work through the contradictions that exist and even recognize those contradictions in the worker's own thinking. This, at least, is the first step toward a society that promotes fair allocation of resources (justice) and individual flourishing (virtue). In recognizing those contradictions the worker will look in two directions: past and future. In looking to past history, it is possible to acknowledge losses, failings, and tragic choices rooted in family dynamics, individual metabolism, economic circumstance, and a thousand other details that circumscribe what it is possible to do for an individual patient in a facility. Judgments of equity—what is "the right thing to do" for the case before me—depend upon that acknowledgment of past history.

At the same time, the social worker must begin to see the pattern by which contradictions unfold in practice: the point made earlier concerning level of action and the distinction between a moral dilemma and a practical problem of implementation. It is a great danger to focus exclusively on micro-problems or micro-dilemmas, just as it is a great danger to allow policy-level or individual-level ethics to "invade" professional judgment. Once we have separated levels of action, it is necessary to correlate them once again and to ask why contradictions arise in the first place: in other words, is this dilemma absolutely necessary? Some of the losses of old age will be unavoidable (bereavement, historical discontinuity, lowered life expectancy, probability of chronic illness, and disability): these are "existential" problems of life. But other late life losses (economic vulnerability, disengagement, loss of meaning) are socially mediated and challenge our sense of social justice.

Long-term care exists in the twilight between unavoidable losses and socially mediated losses. As long as Alzheimer's disease remains incurable and unpreventable, the human tragedy—the unavoidable loss—will exist. If our ideal of social justice challenges the existence of nursing homes, then we must ask in turn, where will these hundreds of thousands of Alzheimer's patients live? Nursing home care—with all of its difficulties—is a "socially mediated loss" but so is indefinite home care for such patients: what some have called the "36-hour day." A recent critic of public policy on nursing homes in America, Bruce Vladeck, favors reducing the institutionalized population, but even he agrees that a large residual population (mainly Alzheimer's) should remain institutionalized. When we contemplate this group of patients we begin to see that abstract principles ("the priority of liberty," a "free market for medical care") are inadequate to cope with the tragic choices that individuals and families must make. Rights, utility, and virtue each have a claim to make in the debate about social justice, but where we draw the line—how many should be institutionalized—will remain a matter of judgment.

Conclusion

"Why are you tormenting me with these unsolved—maybe unsolvable—questions? With all the pain of working in long-term care settings, do we really need this? Finally, if philosophers and moral thinkers over two thousand years haven't been able to solve these problems, why should we pay attention to them now?" The response just cited is an understandable one, but each of these objections puts the whole matter upside-down. The problems themselves—above all, the ones that torment us—are not invented by academicians and philosophers. On the contrary, they are precisely the questions that social workers, and other professionals, talk about, if not in the nursing home dining room, then with their spouses or friends. We pursue the questions because the situations *themselves*, and the decisions that must be made, are tormenting us.

But if they're tormenting us already, why pursue an ethical analysis of such questions? Because we can't help giving reasons for our decisions and we can't avoid the decisions that must be made. Even *not* to decide—for example, on a resident's request to help commit suicide—even this is *already* a decision. And so on for each of the dilemmas that are faced. To avoid talking or thinking about such decisions is one way of coping, but in the long run it is an unsatisfactory style of coping, as any serious reflection on psychology will convince us. Repression and avoidance is not the path to successful coping with such stress as a long-term care setting will be likely to induce. Even if problems cannot be altogether solved, it is essential for a professional's *own* mental health to face the problems head-on, with all the intellectual and emotional resources one commands. One of those intellectual resources is found in the systematic reasoning of moral philosophy and this fact is one of the best reasons for reflecting on ethical dilemmas in long-term care.

But there is a still better reason to mention, and this is in response to the claim that moral philosophy cannot "solve" the problems we face. In one sense, the charge is true, but no more so than it is for medicine. Medicine is not to be rejected because it cannot definitively "solve" the problems of disease and death: that is, the fact that people ultimately grow old and die. But *how* we grow old and die is an all-important challenge. And just as medicine offers some partial, occasionally definitive cures along the way, so the history of moral philosophy shows that *some* problems have been solved, or at least we have learned definitively where the false answers are seen to lie. Knowing wrong answers, detecting fallacies and inadequate arguments: this is not a small achievement and may prove to be a very large contribution to helping professionals cope with painful dilemmas faced in long-term care settings. At least we have no choice but to try. An aging society will increasingly force of all us to face with honesty and courage the final stage of life and the choices that belong to that last stage.

REFERENCES

1. Reamer, Frederic G., & Abramson, Marcia. *The Teaching of Social Work Ethics*, Hastings-on-Hudson, NY: Institute of Society, Ethics, and the Life Sciences, 1982.

2. Preston, Ronald Philip. *The Dilemmas of Care: Social and Nursing Adaptions to the Deformed, the Disabled and the Aged*, New York: Elsevier, 1979.

3. Kohl, Marvin. *Beneficent Euthanasia*, Buffalo, NY: Prometheus Books, 1975.

4. Lewis, Harold. "Morality and the Politics of Practice," *Social Casework*, 1972, Vol. 53, p.p. 404-417.

5. Wilson, Susanna J. *Confidentiality in Social Work*, New York: Free Press, 1978.

6. *Code of Ethics*. New York: National Association of Social Workers, 1980.

7. Rawls, John. *A Theory of Justice*, Cambridge, MA: Harvard University Press, 1971.

Chapter 6

UNDERSTANDING ILLNESS AND AGING

Mildred D. Mailick

Perhaps more than any other age stage in the human life cycle, changes occurring in old age can be best understood within a multi-dimensional, multi-causal framework. The interactive effects of genetics, personality, social situation, role and status deficits, bereavement, isolation, loss of cognitive capacity, reduced income, and illness are difficult, if not impossible, to consider separately. Each has the potential for activating one or more of the others so that the impact of one problem may set off reverberations that may be reflected in all spheres of the individual's functioning. To factor out illness and its impact on the older person is especially difficult since increasing age and illness are not only positively related in the minds of the general public, but their relationship is also documented in epidemiological studies. Chronic illness and disabilities are especially prevalent in old age. Eighty-five percent of the individuals 65 years of age and older report at least one chronic illness. Dental, visual, hearing, and motor impairments also become increasingly common with advancing age.[1]

Within a multi-dimensional framework, some of the ways in which illness and old age interact will be explored in this chapter. Current hypotheses about the causal relationship between illness and old age are briefly surveyed. Two frameworks for examining the impact of illness on the elderly are presented for their utility in informing social work practice.

The Onset of Illness in Old Age

The causes of increased illness in old age have been widely discussed by those doing research in the field of gerontology. Maturational-organic factors are unquestionably important in the development of illness. Genetic

113

theories of aging suggest possible upper limits to the life span caused either by a pre-programmed number of times cell division can take place, or by changes and errors in the DNA molecules. Physiological theories explain limitations in the life span on the basis of a breakdown or dysfunction in one or more of the major organs in the body. Other hypotheses suggest that immunological dysfunction increases with age and leaves the body unable to combat infections or foreign organisms in the system. Autoimmune reactions in which the immune system ceases to distinguish between normal and abnormal cells have also given rise to theories of the relationship of illness and aging. All of these theories and indeed others need further research, but they do offer promise for the future as they suggest ways in which illness and dysfunction may possibly be staved off for longer periods at the end of the life span.[2]

Research suggests that while these biological factors are necessary to the understanding of illness and its relationship to aging, they are not by themselves sufficient. Social and psychological determinants also need to be taken into account so as to explain the variability in the way people respond to both processes. The impact that a wide variety of psychosocial factors have on the health of the aging individual has been extensively studied by social scientists, Binstock, Shanas and others.[3]

The association of psychological factors—personality, psychodynamics, previous life events, and stress—as causal factors of illness is currently being studied, and is still subject to considerable controversy. For example, there is growing interest in the possible effects of depression, hopelessness and grief on the development of cancer as well as the relationship of certain lifelong personality and behavioral characteristics to the incidence of hypertension.[4,5]

Some promising research has been conducted on the connection between stress and the development of chronic illness. Stress may have either a positive or a negative effect, challenging the individual to adapt or overwhelming his or her capacity to respond. Selye and others suggest a process by which prolonged stress in susceptible people may result in physiological changes that lead to illness.[6] More recent epidemiological research conducted by Eisdorfer and Wilkie establishes a significant relationship between the stress engendered by both favorable and negative life changes and the number of illnesses reported in a study population. Life changes causing the most severe stress predicted a higher prevalence of illness.[7]

The association between stressful events and illness has been extensively studied for those under 65. Less research has been conducted on how these factors affect the aged. The meaning of certain stressful events

may be different to those over 65. Neugarten has suggested that li
events such as the death of a spouse that occurs "on time" may not
be as stressful to the older person as it might if it occurred "prematurely"
to someone not psychologically prepared.[8] On the other hand, the physiological response to stress may be different in old age. The elderly have
a greater vulnerability to illness, and small amounts of stress may have
a more severe effect on them than might be the case in a younger
population. Further investigation of this problem is indicated.

Other types of variability in illness response to stressful events in the
lives of the elderly may be explained by the social conditions under
which the elderly live. Social class, culture, status, role, family, and
social support networks are among the many social factors that can affect
what happens to the individual in later life. Constriction of roles—occupational, family and community—are often cited as being associated
with isolation, anomie, poor self-esteem, and failing emotional and physical health. In a study of 4,400 widowers 55 years and older, the incidence of morbidity was sixty-seven percent higher than the general
population of the same age. The relationship between loss of role and
illness has also been demonstrated by studies of separation and divorce,
loss of job and loss of social support systems.[9]

Closely connected to the work on roles is the research on social
support networks. Beginning evidence points to the value of social support groups in mitigating the effect of loss of social role. Social support
networks provide personal contact, emotional support, information and
material aid to the elderly person. Case studies and other research reports emphasize the importance of family and other networks in the maintenance of health and the reduction in the susceptibility to illness in
the elderly.[10]

Factors in the socioeconomic structure are of equal importance. In
general, the lower the socioeconomic status, the higher the prevalence
of disease among the elderly.[11] While a specific causal relationship between low income and the incidence of illness has been difficult to
establish, it is clear that access to environmental resources is easier
for those with higher income and may be an important predictor of the
ability of the chronically ill person to be sustained in the community.

The Impact of Illness

Thus, the incidence of illness rises in the elderly under conditions
in which physiological, emotional, and social deprivations converge.
Similarly, once illness strikes, many factors act together to affect how the

l responds. It is difficult to predict which factors will
ient ones and the most important in any single case. The
)f each person's life history, the capacity which is built
pan for coping with and defending against adversity as
... u₃ the level of emotional and physical stamina all must be taken
into account. Resources in the family and community for providing services and the nature and severity of the specific illness are additional
factors to be considered. As yet, no single overall frame of reference has
been developed that has provided sufficient predictive capacity. Rather,
each of the various theoretical approaches help to provide separate pieces
in the patchwork of understanding the impact of chronic illness on the
aged. Several will be examined for their possible utility in understanding
aspects of the functioning of the aged individual coping with serious
acute or chronic illness.

Psychodynamic Factors in Illness

Each aged person faces some fairly universal experiences and tasks
which are related to the final stage of life. These include adapting to
losses and decrements of various kinds, reorganizing aspirations, self-
image and time perspective and engaging in a reassessment and acceptance of the existential meaning of one's own life. How the individual
responds to the experiences and resolves the tasks is dependent partially
on the capacity of the ego to meet the demands and to maintain the
balance and integrity of ego boundaries.

With the onset of illness, the demands on the ego are intensified as
the aged individual must respond not only to the usual tasks of aging, but
also to those imposed by the illness. Coping and defense patterns, successful in early life, may be weakened by the convergence of the two.
The individual strives to maintain psychic integrity in the face of the
depletion of resources. Cath suggests that developmental vulnerabilities
and arrests become more significant as the individual regresses, reversing
the order in which the personality was formed.[12] By this process, relations
with the superego and especially with ego ideals are most likely to be
the first to undergo change. The gradual relinquishment of expectations
for the self which are no longer realistic is a normal task of old age.
However, when the ego is placed under the dual stress of the aging process
and the impact of illness, the painful struggle is intensified. Pain, dis-
figurement, immobility, and other effects of illness may overwhelm the
healthier defenses of the individual and bring into play more primitive

ones in an effort to relinquish no longer realistic goals and still maintain self-esteem.

Other superego functions are also affected by the defense of regression. Unacceptable feelings, normally controlled by the superego, may become conscious and be expressed. Since the process of regression leaves parts of the superego intact, the elderly person may experience overwhelming guilt at the expression of aggression and rage. Illness increases guilt at the same time that it constricts the number of healthy outlets for the expression of feeling. Rage, guilt and depression are a common triad, followed eventually by apathy.

Regression of the ego may also follow a reverse epigenetic course. Object relations may take on more primitive forms with the withdrawal of cathexis from the external world and reinvestment in self. Some turning inward is adaptive to the process of aging, although it is not clear whether increasing interiority occurs independently or in response to a rejecting environment. The onset of illness may evoke a more severe withdrawal which is maladaptive, eventuating in excessive concern with the self, hypochrondriacal fears and possible delusions.

Changes in other aspects of object relations are commonly noted among the elderly. Relationships with others may become symbiotic, either more dependent or more domineering, depending on the individual situation. Under the stress of illness, object relations may deteriorate even further. Splitting may take place, as can be seen when the elderly individual perceives adult children and/or health care professionals as either good or bad objects.

The organization of the defense mechanisms may undergo similar regressive changes. Defenses most central to the individual's character structure are likely to remain intact while those adopted more recently are likely to be less stable. Illness brings with it a feeling of anxiety, helplessness and vulnerability and can activate denial, projection and other primitive defenses developed early in life.

The most crucial task of the ego when facing the dual stress of old age and illness is the attempt to maintain self-esteem. The importance of narcissism in maintaining self-esteem even when assaulted by losses, is discussed by Kohut.[13] People draw self-esteem from a variety of sources. Some of it is internalized during the early developmental stages and the remainder is derived from positively cathected object relations, ongoing adult role and status gratifications, creativity, successful achievement, and a variety of activities.[14] Physical debilitation, loss of attractiveness, isolation, loss of roles and activities occasioned by illness all can impair and assault the feelings of self-esteem. Vulnerability to loss of self-esteem is especially acute when the particular sources of gratification most positively cathected are no longer available. An example is the elderly man or woman for whom body image and physical capacity are crucial to self-esteem and who through sudden loss of these by virtue of illness or various types of treatments such as surgery or chemotherapy experiences a loss of a sense of their own body integrity.

The importance of early childhood in the development of healthy narcissism has been repeatedly emphasized by Cath, Mahler and others. The child internalizes the admiration, pleasure and responsiveness to need of the caretaking adults, resolves feelings of omnipotence and grandiosity and is left with an enduring, positive feeling about the self. This reservoir of healthy narcissism is available for emotional refueling when external sources are constricted. It is this inner strength that is drawn on by the aging individual, especially during periods of object loss and illness. The capacity to draw on inner resources during periods of loss may be the critical source in maintaining ego integrity and the motivation to recoup, to recathect to new objects and to find other sources of gratification.

Changes in the impulses are affected by aging and illness. Although some individuals maintain functional genital sexuality into late old age, others do not. Differences in sex role behavior of men and women narrow in old age. Regression to a pre-genital sexuality can be adaptive especially to those elderly who, through attenuation of impulse, loss of partner, or physical incapacity, no longer seek intercourse. Sexuality, however, can continue to be an important source of gratification and self-esteem. A normal aging process allows for the broadening of the range of gratification through other forms of sexuality such as touching and holding. However, illness may complicate this positive adaptation if the individual is conflicted or has remnants of guilt about the expression of sexuality. The illness may also be consciously or unconsciously perceived as retaliation for sexual fantasies, impulses and activities not acceptable to a harsh superego and thus may impel repression or reaction formations of various sorts. The expression of aggression is also complicated for the ill elderly person who may have increased dependency needs. Relationship with family members and others are fraught with fear of loss of support if normal assertiveness is exercised. The sick role may be used to attempt to legitimize releasing aggression through complaints and demands.

In sum, all three structural systems of the personality, the superego,

ego and id, may be affected by the interactive effects of illness and old age. The course of regression in any of the systems is seldom uniform and pockets of more mature functions can exist along with more primitive forms. The unevenness is important to keep in mind as it may provide potential for intervention. While the concept of total cure is incompatible to both the problems of the ill elderly and to social work intervention, there is much that can be done to help the individual maintain integrity of the personality. Assistance can be provided in reassessing and re-organizing expectations of self, reducing anguish about giving up roles and activities that can no longer be performed and freeing some of the guilt that accompanies old age and illness. Educative and supportive intervention can also encourage expression of impulses in ways that are compatible with the individual's culture, life history and personal situation. If self-image is considered the crucial factor in maintaining ego integrity, then sensitive and careful supportive work can augment narcissistic refueling and encourage a process of recathecting with re-parative external objects and activities.

Social Psychological Approach

The psychodynamic approach provides a close look at the intrapsychic factors that might be affected by age and illness. It emphasizes the uniqueness of each individual. The combinations of intrapsychic forces are almost unlimited so that no two people respond to the impact of illness in the same way. Yet it is helpful to take a broader perspective and to group together people with similarity of response so that their essential uniformity rather than their uniqueness can contribute to the understanding of the impact of illness. Many groupings have been pro-posed by social psychologists and tested by research. One approach that has potential for describing the impact of illness on the elderly was proposed by research which was undertaken by David Guttman of the Committee on Human Development of the University of Chicago.[15] Developed and tested on a group of 145 mentally and physically well men of 40 to 70 years of age, it grouped the men into three main categories according to the way in which they seemed to master both internal and external problems. The groups were called "Active Mastery," "Passive Mastery," and "Magical Mastery."

The research was repeated and the categories were validated as ex-isting in other cultural groups as well. However, the categories may not be generalizable to women, to minority sub-cultures, or to all classes within society without further validation. It does provide an interesting framework for analyzing possible responses by the aged to the impact of illness.

The *Active Mastery* group is described as alloplastic in their orientation, valuing their own autonomy, competence and capacity to control the external environment. They are uncomfortable with dependency or having to comply to the wishes of others. They deny internal conflict by projection and externalization. Not introspective themselves they are more concerned about the behavior than the intentions of others. This coping style is adaptive if the individual is physically well, relatively young and in control of environmental resources, but poses obvious problems to the ill and the elderly. An aged individual with an active mastery orientation is more likely to ignore physical symptoms and when no longer able to do so, to deny their possible serious implications. Such a person may attempt self-medication rather than place themselves in the hands of the physician. When forced to seek medical attention by advancing illness, they will try to control as much of the process as possible. They often refuse to accept diagnosis, especially if it requires surgery or other invasive treatments. Their tendency to project tends to make them difficult patients as they defend against feelings of fear and rage by exhibiting distrust, especially by questioning the competence of medical personnel. Physical deficits and incapacities attack their central source of self-esteem—their sense of autonomy and their ability to control their own lives. Loss of control of bodily functions and the need for help in continuing to live massively threatens those with this coping orientation. Those who are most rigid in their personality organization are emotionally at highest risk in the last stage of life. Their tendency to see themselves in an adversary position to their environment makes accepting advancing frailty and incapacity insupportably humiliating. Those with healthier personalities may use their coping strength to deal with their illness and incapacity as a challenge. They attempt to control as much of their environment as they can in order to protect their inner sense of competence. While they may have to relinquish partial or complete control of their bodies to the care of others, their inner standards for themselves may become their principal challenge. Their effort to die with dignity is the final expression of their style of mastery.

The *Passive Mastery* group is described as autoplastic in orientation. They tend to accommodate themselves to the external world, regarding the environment as powerful and unpredictable. They adjust to what others expect in order to gain acceptance and indulgence. Actively avoiding conflict, constricting opportunities and new experiences, they value internal security rather than external mastery and control. They have traded autonomy and the expressions of individuality in order to receive protection from dangerous outside forces.

Illness represents an undeserved retribution meted out in spite of efforts to conform and be accepted. It is perceived as being imposed by external forces and the expectation is that through the care they receive from others, they will be helped to get better. On the surface those with a passive mastery coping style make good patients. Conditioned to looking to powerful others for protection and nurturance, they tend to consult physicians relatively soon after symptoms develop, accept diagnoses and comply with treatment recommendations meticulously. If hospitalized, they try not to "bother" the nurses, fearing that if they do, they may not be attended to when they really need assistance.[16] Being taken care of meets their most basis needs, and illness legitimates demands for nurturance and protection. Underneath this compliance, however, is an unspoken demand: conformity and agreeableness brings with it the expectation of caring and curing. The responsibility for getting well may subtly shift from the patient to the physician or other health care professionals. The patient expects that the physician will effect a cure or at least make every effort to alleviate pain and discomfort through the use of medication and other ameliorative treatments. When illness brings severe pain and disability to this group, they tend to become childlike, wanting increasing attention and care. Their major concern is not the challenge of death with dignity, but drawing on resources so as not to die alone or in pain.

Those with *Magical Mastery* comprise the third group. Unlike the other two groups, neither alloplastic nor autoplastic efforts are made to control the environment which is seen as dangerous and capricious. Instrumental action is considered useless and therefore delay in gratification unnecessary. Reality testing is poor, and fantasy and wish fulfillment are confused with actuality. Primitive defense mechanisms such as denial and projection are most commonly used. When the magical mastery group become ill, they see their situation as further evidence of the capriciousness of fate or other supernatural forces. They ignore symptoms as long as possible, hoping that somehow they will disappear. Before consulting physicians, they are likely to try magical or ritual/religious cures for illnesses, especially if these are syntonic with their cultural or religious beliefs. When they do seek medical care, they expect that the physician will follow certain rituals (give them a physical examination, provide a specific diagnosis and prescribe some medication). Their need for immediate gratification causes poor compliance with medical regimens. They do not consistently follow instructions, often ceasing to take medications before they should and failing to adhere to dietary and other restrictions. They tend to have difficult relationships with physicians to whom they either ascribe omnipotent power or perceive as threatening hostile objects. They may not be conscious of their rage and fear at being ill, projecting these feelings onto others. Helpless to deal either actively on their own behalf, or passively by manipulation, they feel vulnerable and at the mercy of others. As death approaches, the more emotionally vulnerable of them may become delusional while the better adapted ones may be comforted by denial, magical thinking and by resigning themselves to fate or religion.

Thus, each of the three groups responds to illness in distinctive ways. Intervention can be more effectively provided if coping styles can be identified and supported by flexible provision of health care and other services. While these are styles of mastery that can be useful, categorizing people within them does not obviate the necessity of then individualizing each person within the group and responding so as to provide for his or her own unique needs.

Research suggests that a significantly larger number of men 60 years and older were found to use Magical Mastery as a method of coping than did younger men. Health care professionals are probably most uncomfortable with this orientation. In a culture where instrumentality is highly valued, it is difficult for them to appreciate adaptive potentials of a Magical Mastery orientation. The problems of aging, illness, failing strength, restricted mobility and cognitive capacity, and the existential closeness of death may force a reorganization of the ego in old age in which rationality and instrumentality seem less appropriate than delivering oneself into the hands of fate. Health care professionals should strive to help keep the individual as active and instrumental as possible, but should also be sensitive to shifts in orientation which may be important to accept and support.

Neither the psychodynamic nor the social psychological frameworks which have been presented adequately explains the impact of illness on the aged. Each of these approaches is mediated by environmental factors. In fact, some researchers suggest that it is the environmental factors that form the independent variables with personality factors constituting intervening contingencies in the prediction of response to illness in old age. In any case, it is important to take into account the interaction between the personality and the environment in understanding the impact of illness on the aging process.

The elderly individual is best understood within his or her natural context in which functional relationships can be assessed, taking into account all the salient human and non-human systems. Such a broadened framework recognizes the importance of the cultural, social and economic elements and extends its focus to the effects of patterns of service, organizational and institutional behavior, and even spatial and geographic factors. Not all of these components are considered in every case; rather only those directly relevant to the situation of the aged individual are included. In some, intrapsychic and intrafamilial components are most important, but in others different social support networks, social service and health agencies, and physical space may need to be included. Each component that is considered becomes part of a transactional matrix. Intervention occurs in any part of the matrix that has potential for helping the elderly person maintain ego integrity and maximum functional capacity within the limits of the illness.

The dimensions of this framework encompass varied levels of conceptualization. Medicine, psychiatry, sociology, anthropology, psychology, architecture, urban planning, and political science all contribute substance to this interdisciplinary approach. The point of conceptual convergence is their relationship to the elderly individual. The use of this broadened framework provides social workers giving services to the elderly with an opportunity to view problems of the aged through lenses that transcend traditional disciplinary boundaries. It has the potential for creating new understanding of the impact of illness on the aged and this can lead to new methods of intervention.

Implications for Intervention

Assessment

Assessment of the elderly ill person is a complex task that often involves a collaborative effort involving physicians, nurses, social workers, physical therapists, psychiatrists, and other health givers. It should reflect all areas of functioning of the older person. Distinctions between the effects of aging and the effects of illness can be critical in establishing a plan of service. At times, the symptoms of the older person are attributed to the irreversible forces of aging and therapeutic activities are not pursued actively enough. A careful assessment may reveal many spheres in which prompt attention will lead to a stabilization or reversal of symptoms and improvement in functioning.

Social work assessment includes relevant data about the individual's life history, former methods of coping, current strengths and capacities to persevere in spite of illness and advancing disability, functional capacities, level of motivation and emotional as well as physical stamina. The psychodynamic framework of assessment contributes to an understanding of the individual's inner resources. Knowledge about the individual's characteristic style of mastery helps to establish clues to providing service in ways that are compatible with the life-style of the individual. Assessment of family and environmental resources are of equal importance. Family and other support networks must be realistically considered. Understanding the way in which the elderly person fits into the life of the family may be decisive in providing a workable plan for the older person. Knowledge about the availability of appropriate community services that can support the elderly ill person and the family form a critical part of the assessment process.

Intervention

The social worker has a broad spectrum of interventive strategies at his or her disposal that can be employed to help the elderly person deal with the effects of illness and aging. As with other population groups, the social work objective is to help the individual achieve as full a realization of potential as possible within the limitations imposed by the illness and the environment.

More than any other life stage, the needs of the elderly ill client are likely to be multifaceted, requiring a combination of environmental, interpersonal and intrapsychic interventions. Survival needs must be met first. The quality of life for some elderly people erodes slowly, and their housing, heat and amenities often deteriorate gradually without their envisaging the possibility of change. Similarly, inadequate food and clothing are endured. It is often during the crisis of illness that these inadequately met needs become evident, and attending to them is an important part of social work treatment. As with any intervention the attempt is made to provide appropriate services that reflect the client's right to exercise choice and is supportive of their style of mastery and self-esteem.

Intervention with family and others who give care has the goal of helping to maintain their capacity to provide a reliable source of physical and emotional support to the elderly individual. The social worker can often be instrumental in helping the family to balance its own needs for gratification, individuation and growth and yet remain a resource of the elderly person. Sometimes when family members are freed of guilt for what they cannot give, they can offer some emotional support and services. These need to be supplemented with community services as available and appropriate. Every effort should be made to preserve communication and interaction with family members and other social support networks.

All aspects of work with the elderly person should be focused on helping them to maintain their self-esteem. The losses that take place with illness and old age deprive the individual of lifelong sources of narcissistic gratification. While capacity to withstand pain and loss caused by old age and illness is, at least partially dependent on an inner reservoir of narcissism that is laid down in early childhood, those who lack this endowment can be helped to avoid retreat into excessive preoccupation with themselves. These individuals need support in overcoming isolation and in recathecting with new objects. New activities that are within the capacities of the elderly ill person may supply fresh sources of support of self-esteem and status. The critical therapeutic effort is to help the individual shift their own expectations of self so that they are not continually depleted by their sense of loss of capacity to be loved. The social worker can be of decisive importance in this endeavor not only by direct supportive treatment, but also by encouraging significant others to reinforce this acceptance of revised expectations. The individual must be helped to value continued capacities rather than dwell on those things that he or she can no longer do or be. Reactivating the individual's self-esteem has the potential of creating a reverberating circuit as it leads to improved functioning and thus to greater positive feedback from the external environment.

Intervention on behalf of the elderly ill person requires many services which may not be available within one agency. The social worker is often called upon to develop a package of services, coordinating them on behalf of the client and working collaboratively with other professionals. When services are not available, case and class advocacy and political action are a part of social work practice.

In summary, competent, consistent and timely social work intervention can be of pivotal importance in working with the elderly population. The social work knowledge and values which underpin the assessment and interventive process support a multi-faceted biopsychosocial approach.

This expanded view of practice can help people pursue maximum potential in the last stage of life.

REFERENCES

1. Shanas, Ethel and Maddox, George. "Aging, Health and the Organization of Health Resources," *Handbook of Aging and the Social Sciences*, edited by Robert H. Binstock and Ethel Shanas, New York: Van Nostrand Reinhold Company, 1976.
2. Shock, Nathan. "Biological Theories of Aging," *Handbook of the Psychology of Aging*, edited by James E. Birren and K. Warner Schaie, New York: Van Nostrand Reinhold Company, 1977.
3. Binstock, Robert and Shanas, Ethel, editors. *Handbook of Aging and the Social Sciences, op. cit.*
4. Sklar, Lawrence S. and Anisman, Hymie. "Stress and Cancer," *Psychological Bulletin* 89:3, (1981), pp. 369-406.
5. Eisdorfer, Carl and Wilkie, Frances, "Stress, Disease, Aging and Behavior," in *Handbook of the Psychology of Aging, op. cit.*, pp. 251-275.
6. Selye, Hans. "Stress and Aging," *Journal of the American Geriatric Society*, 18:660-681, (1970).
7. Eisdorfer, & Wilkie, *op. cit.*
8. Neugarten, Bernice and Hagestad, Gunhild. "Age and the Life Course," in Binstock, *Handbook of Aging and Social Sciences, op. cit.* pp. 35-55.
9. Pilisuk, Marc and Minkler, Meredith. "Supportive Networks: Life Ties for the Elderly," *Journal of Social Issues* 36:2, (1980), pp. 95-115.
10. Pilisuk, & Minkler, *op. cit.*
11. Shanas, & Maddox, *op. cit.*
12. Cath, Stanley. "Suicide in the Middle Years: Some Reflections on the Annihilation of Self," in Mid-Life Developmental and Clinical Issues edited by William Norman and Thomas Scaramella, New York: Brunner Mazel, 1980, pp. 53-72.
13. Kohut, Heinz. *The Restoration of the Self*, New York: International University Press, 1977, pp.116-117.
14. Cath, Stanley, *op. cit.*
15. Gutmann. *The Country of Old Men: Cultural Studies in the Psychology of Later Life*, Ann Arbor, Michigan: Institute of Gerontology, University of Michigan, 1969.
16. Tagliacozzo, Daisy and Mauksch, Hans. "The Patient's View of the Patient's Role," *Patients, Physicians and Illness*, edited by E. Gartly Jaco, Second Edition, New York: Free Press, 1972, pp. 162-175.

Chapter 7

SOCIOCULTURAL DIMENSIONS: NURSING HOMES AND THE MINORITY AGED

Barbara Jones Morrison

Introduction

This chapter will examine the role which ethnic and cultural factors play in long-term care service delivery to aged persons from racial and ethnic minority groups.* Several dimensions will be addressed, including sociocultural determinants of (1) risk and need of institutional long-term care, (2) patterns of long-term care utilization by minority group aged, and (3) provider and consumer attitudes with respect to design and delivery of services to minority aged.

In recent years comparative data on different aged racial or ethnic cohorts have become more available, although large-scale nationally representative data sets are rare. In the past gerontological research studies were likely not to include racial or ethnic minority aged in their samples and if they did, important variables were rarely disaggregated by age and race or ethnicity simultaneously. Research on minorities in long-term care settings is even more limited than research on community-based populations. Fortunately, a few ground breaking studies have been undertaken on this topic in recent years.[1] The purpose of this chapter will be to use the findings from recent studies of minorities in long-term care to define and illustrate the ways in which racial or ethnic factors influence the design and utilization of institutional long-term care, thereby deriving some generalizable principles to guide practice.

---

*The term "minority aged" in this paper refers to aged persons from non-white ethnic groups. Illustrative examples are derived from studies examining long-term care for aged blacks, Asian-Americans, Hispanics and American Indians.

Sociocultural Determinants of Risk and Need

Research on the institutionalized aged population has shown the consistent emergence of three factors which are predictive of the need for long-term institutional care. The first is deteriorating physical and mental health: 80% of the institutionalized aged have serious health problems or impaired mental functioning. An inability to perform the basic activities of daily living with concomitant limited mobility is frequently observed. The second is advanced age: more than half of the institutionalized aged population is over 80 years of age and the chances of becoming institutionalized increase with age. The third factor is marital and family status: there are three times as many widowed persons in long-term care facilities as there are married or single individuals. Many more aged in institutions never had children or outlived their children as compared to aged still residing in the community.[2]

To the extent that racial, ethnic or cultural factors influence patterns of health, longevity and marital or family status, one would expect racial or ethnic minority aged to display a different pattern of risk and need for institutional long-term care compared to white aged.

If health status were the sole risk factor, aged from minority groups would be at greater risk. There is ample evidence to indicate that compared to whites of comparable ages, non-white aged have poorer self-reported health status, as well as observable increases in the number of chronic and disabling health conditions.

For example, a 1980 report on *Characteristics of the Black Elderly*[3] stated that based on several measures, older blacks appear to suffer more from the effects of chronic health conditions and other illnesses and injuries than whites in the same age group. Using data from the *National Center for Health Statistics*, the report goes on to note that 51% of blacks 65 years and older were limited in their ability to perform major activities such as working and the tasks of daily living due to chronic impairments as compared to 36% of whites age 65 and older. One fourth (27%) of blacks in this age group were entirely unable to carry on routine tasks as compared to 16% of their white counterparts. Persons of black and other races were 57% more likely than comparable whites to be confined to their houses because of chronic impairments.[4]

In a Los Angeles based study of 1,269 white, black and Mexican-American elderly, Dowd and Bengston[5] found that minority aged were in poorer health compared to whites at each age stratum with the greatest disparity occurring among those aged 65 years and older. Cantor[6] reported similar findings in her study of New York City's elderly population.

Income level and socioeconomic status appear to be related to health status for all age groups, including the elderly. Poverty is associated with poorer health throughout the life cycle and decreased longevity. The greater incidence of poverty among minority groups means that they are more likely to die at younger ages as Dowd and Bengston indicate:

> While it is possible that poorer health reported by the minority aged may reflect a bio-genetical difference between whites and non-whites that is also manifest in the different life expectancies at birth for each group, the more probable explanation for these health differences is a sociological one. Because of past and present policies of racial discrimination in our society, non-whites have had less income, inadequate nutrition and, consequently poorer health and a lower life expectancy at birth than whites.[7]

The lower life expectancies of minority aged, and minority aged males in particular, decreases their risk of institutionalization. Based on 1977 demographic data, life expectancy at birth for "Blacks and other races" was 64.6 years for males and 73.1 years for females. Comparable figures for whites were 70 years for males and 77.7 years for females. The predominance of white females among the residents of long-term care facilities is directly related to their increased longevity relative to other groups.

Eribes and Bradley-Rawls refer to observed life expectancy differentials among racial or ethnic groups as the "biogenetic" hypothesis for explaining differential risk of institutionalization for non-whites.[8] In their study of elderly Mexican-Americans in the Southwest, they examined life expectancy tables for the Spanish-surnamed population in Arizona (one of the few states, they noted, to collect birth and death statistics separately for the Spanish-surnamed population). Life expectancy for the Spanish-surnamed population was 67.2 years—a 4.1 year diference from whites in the area who could expect to live to age 71.

Life expectancy tables reveal another demographic trend which may hold implications for an increased need of institutional long-term care by minority aged in the future. This phenomenon, referred to by demographers as the "cross-over" effect, has been consistently observed. Men of black and other races who do reach age 65 (and remember that they represent a minority), tend to live longer than their white counterparts, with the greatest cross-over occurring after age 80. Women of black and other races who live to age 75 tend to outlive their white counterparts.[9] Although these "super survivors" are not great in absolute numbers, a continuation of this trend in the future will see a growth in the number of very old minority aged who may increase the demand for institutional long-term care.

On the factors of marital and family status a mixed pattern of risk emerges. It is perhaps in this domain that specific ethnic groups differ most and where the confounding effects of social class position are greatest. In general the view is held that non-white aged are less at risk of institutionalization because they are relatively advantaged compared to whites with respect to availability of family to care for them in times of prolonged illness or incapacity. Availability of spouse or adult children who can assume caretaking responsibilities is not uniform across ethnic groups or within ethnic groups. Black elderly, for example, are as likely as whites to have been married at some point in their lives, however, they are less likely to enter old age still married. Rubenstein[10] reported that one out of every five black elderly women are living apart from their husbands. In addition, black women are at much greater risk of early widowhood when the marriage does survive because of the lower life expectancy of black males. These patterns were especially true of older blacks in urban areas.

Among New York City's urban elderly, Cantor found that black women had the second highest rate of marriage, but only 29% were still married at the time of the study. When compared to white and Hispanic aged, blacks had the highest rates of divorce and separation.[11]

Although a spouse may not always be available, black and other minority aged appear to be advantaged with respect to availability of children to provide care when needed. Minority women have traditionally had more children than their white counterparts. They consequently enter old age with larger family networks. References to the "extended family" abound in the literature on minority groups. The prevalence of the extended family among minority groups is changing—at least as far as the traditional multigenerational household is concerned. Current research indicates that extended family arrangements and relationships vary by a number of sociodemographic variables including ethnicity (i.e., more prevalent among Hispanics than whites or blacks); geography (i.e., more prevalent in rural and core inner-city areas); social class position (i.e., more prevalent among the lower classes); immigration status (i.e., more prevalent among recent arrivals) and sex of the aged parent (i.e., more prevalent when the aged parent in the extended household is a woman).[12]

Currently and increasingly so in the future, minority family structures will be changing because of social and economic pressures which impact all other American families. Notable among these pressures will be the unprecedented entry of women into the labor force, meaning that women in the family who have traditionally provided "hands-on" care of dependent children and elderly will be less available. The increase in divorce, coupled with the decision by many people to delay or forego marriage and childbearing, to either live alone or in an alternate lifestyle, will mean that traditional family-based caring arrangements will likely change for many groups, including racial and ethnic minority groups. The ultimate impact of these changes for care of the aged in the future is yet to be determined, but effects due to changing social patterns are certainly inevitable.

Sociocultural Determinants of Long-Term Care Utilization

Although the number of institutional long-term care facilities has increased in recent years, their utilization by minority aged has never been great. It has already been noted that decreased longevity and the greater availability of care-taking relatives for some minority aged explain this to some extent. There are, however, a number of other hypotheses which appear in the literature to explain the underutilization of institutional long-term care by racial and ethnic minorities. Data from the 1974 *Minority Health Chartbook*,[13] show that the majority of the nursing homes in the United States do not have minority residents. Forty-two percent reported serving aged blacks, 23.5% had Spanish-surnamed residents, 9% served aged Asian-Americans and 8% had aged American Indians among their resident populations.

In their 1977 DHEW-contracted study of "Special Needs of Racial/Ethnic Minorities and Provider Attitudes in Long-Term Care Facilities,"[14] Forward Management Associates, Inc. interviewed 25 long-term care facility administrators from geographic areas with high density minority populations. In the report they state:

Without exception, the overwhelming reason attributed to the lack of participation by minority groups by long-term care administrators was that black and other minority groups did not like institutionalization and preferred to stay in their accustomed surroundings as long as possible. In as much as there is some basis for this in fact, its ready acceptance may obscure the fact that other factors may be important and contributory.[15]

Support for the "cultural aversion" hypothesis was also found by Morrison in her study of Black Aged in Nursing Homes[16] and by Forward Management Associates Inc. in their national study of ethnic minorities in long-term care.[17]

Assuming that minority families prefer to "care for their own," a critical issue is the extent to which they possess material resources, time, and stamina to care for frail aged members. Perhaps the facile acceptance of the "cultural aversion" hypothesis should be tempered by some empirical evidence on how minority families are taking care of the frail aged with some realistic assessment of costs in both financial and psychosocial terms.

Minority aged who are not in immediate family situations are more at risk of institutionalization. In her study of 93 aged blacks in voluntary nursing homes in New York City, Morrison found that the sex of the older person was significantly related to availability of family, and the role which family played in the placement decision-making process. Black aged males were less likely to have family available to them. Where a family did exist, males were more likely to have been estranged from family members at some earlier point in their lives. Many had been institutionalized without the family's knowing that placement had occurred. Although relationships between female residents and their family members were somewhat better, good family relationships and close affectional ties were not enough to prevent many placements when the demands for 24-hour physical care became too great. The most frequently cited reasons for admission among minority residents was rapidly decreasing physical health coupled with inability of families to manage care any longer.

The important issue here seems to be the danger in overselling the "cultural aversion" hypothesis by both providers and minority group members themselves. The easy and unquestioning acceptance of this view will result in a denial of service to minority aged and their families who may subscribe to the cultural value of "caring for one's own" but lack the capacity to act on that value without significant assistance from the formal service system. Clearly many more community-based supportive services such as home-health assistance, delivered meals and respite care are needed in minority neighborhoods to help families and to delay or mitigate unnecessary placements. However, for many severely incapacitated minority aged the intermediary or skilled long-term care facility represents the better plan of care.

There is always the danger that providers will rely on the preference of minority groups to "care for their own" as a rationalization for lack of outreach and service provision. On the other hand, minority families may too quickly dismiss consideration of the nursing home as a viable plan of care. Because of the strong cultural prescriptions against institutional placements among several ethnic groups, minority families contemplating placement of an aged family member may need special counselling to resolve the value conflicts.

Another hypothesis used to explain the underutilization of nursing homes by minority aged relates to geographic location of most nursing homes vis-à-vis minority communities.

Downing and Copeland have described a number of factors which they believe affect service utilization among aged blacks. Agency location and visibility are two such factors. In their view agencies located within the black community create a warm and favorable climate, whereas those outside the community tend to create ambivalence and suspicion as to their availability to black clients.[18]

Eribes and Bradley-Rawls make reference to the "territorial orientation" of older Mexican-Americans. They cite the work of Orleans (1967), which used cognitive mapping experiments with Mexican-Americans. The results demonstrated the close attachment of the Mexican-American to pedestrian scale neighborhoods, as well as their cognitive inability to perceive or utilize urban facilities and services outside of their closely circumscribed neighborhoods.[19]

Utilization of nursing homes located within minority neighborhoods by minority aged is higher than utilization of facilities located outside minority neighborhoods. Both Morrison and FMA found this to be true of utilization of nursing homes in Central Harlem and Brooklyn by black aged.[20] Of the nursing homes in the FMA sample which served American Indian aged, the greatest utilization was found at the facility located on the Gila Indian Reservation in Phoenix, Arizona.[21] Eribes and Bradley-Rawls reported a slight increase in the percentage of older Mexican-Americans residing within nursing homes located in Mexican-American communities.[22]

The location factor in determining utilization of long-term care facilities by minority aged appears to be a significant one. Location of facilities within minority neighborhoods is typically associated with minority sponsorship of the facility and substantial minority group sponsorship of the facility and substantial minority group representation on the administrative and direct care staff. These elements may also account for increased utilization. One implication of these findings is the need to build more long-term intermediary and skilled nursing facilities within or close to areas where large numbers of minority aged and their families reside. This, however, is a longer range solution to meeting needs. For the present, many minority aged have to be placed in long-term care facilities outside of their accustomed environments. Wherever possible, the best match between the resident's needs and the facility's services should be sought. The ability to achieve this match will depend largely on the adequacy of information and referral services for minority aged and their families with regard to the long-term care delivery system.

The vast majority of referrals to nursing homes for minority aged are made by hospital staff.[23] With the increased emphasis on certification of health status and degree of impairment as criteria for admission, hospital personnel have become more involved in placement decisions.

Nursing home administrators have expressed their belief that not enough information is being given to minority families or aged persons with respect to the location of facilities or the services which they have to offer.[24] Another hypothesis, then, for the underutilization of nursing homes by minority aged is the lack of adequate information and referral services within hospitals and service agencies.

FMA found one example in their field research of the benefits of providing essential information and coordinating the referral and placement process. They describe a program undertaken by a Boston nursing home and Boston City Hospital in which the nursing home's services were well explained to patients in the hospital who would need post-hospitalization care. The referral and admission process was carefully coordinated by the hospital and nursing home staff. Acceptance of the nursing home as a viable alternative was observed to be high by the majority of residents, most of whom were black.[25]

Another problem in the referral process mentioned by some non-white administrators of long-term care facilities was their belief that hospital staff often referred non-white aged to predominantly white facilities because they were perceived to be of better quality.[26] One might expect that there are also those hospital and social agency staff who make referrals only to those facilities which are predominantly non-white on the assumption that minority aged would prefer to be in such facilities. The assumptions which underlie both approaches need to be tested against more information on what constitutes "quality care," as well as the expressed preferences of minority aged consumers.

Finally, economic factors have been related to long-term care utilization by minority aged. The relationships between income, cost of care and utilization of services is a complex one and not well understood. One hypothesis is that as minority group families move up the social and economic ladder, they will make greater use of institutional care for their aged members since the opportunity costs for family-rendered care are greater (e.g., income lost to the wife who stays home to provide care) and the financial costs of care are more within their means.

Eribes and Bradley-Rawls did not find support for this hypothesis among Mexican-Americans. They report a negative association between income and nursing home utilization: as family income rose, nursing home utilization declined. Their conclusion was that it is unlikely that Mexican-American families will increase their utilization of nursing homes as they become better able to afford the cost of institutional care.[27] They also found that as the number of poor Mexican-American aged increased, so did the number of nursing home placements. Over half of the variance in nursing home utilization in this study was explained by the number of older Mexican-Americans below the poverty line.[28]

To some extent the relationship between poverty and nursing home utilization can be explained by differences in health status between poor and non-poor minority aged. Perhaps poverty which as noted before creates lifetime patterns of ill-health creates a greater demand for institutional care in old age. Another important factor is the advent of Medicaid and Medicare which removed financial barriers to long-term care facilities for substantial numbers of aged poor, regardless of race or ethnicity. About 90% of the minority aged in long-term care facilities have the cost of their care paid through Medicaid or similar public systems.[29]

Identification of economic factors which work as either incentives or disincentives to nursing home placement is a fruitful area for more research, specifically with reference to racial and ethnic minorities. It would also be important to ascertain the degree to which minority aged and their families are aware of the availability of public monies like Medicaid to underwrite the costs of nursing home care. Availability of financial assistance would be an important part of the information and referral process, since many families may believe that they must assume the entire cost of care.

The sociocultural factors which appear to be related to both patterns of need and service utilization are many. It is unlikely that any one factor predominates. Like other types of human behavior, nursing home utilization by minority aged is multi-causal and the predictive power of any specific combination of factors may vary, depending on the particular ethnic group one is working with.

After the decision to place has been made, cultural issues become even more salient. Critics of nursing homes have pointed to the lack of a "home-like" quality in these facilities which look like and function like extended care hospitals, for the most part. FMA's report states that "assuming effective delivery of long-term care to be based not only on the medical model, but a creative medical-psychosocial approach, it should become evident that culture, language, dietary and other special factors must be considered in the resident's plan of care."[30]

The remainder of this chapter will be devoted to sociocultural factors to be considered in the design and delivery of institutional long-term care to minority aged. Attitudes of both providers and consumers on the importance of cultural congruence in programming, staffing and decision-making will be explored.

Sociocultural Factors in Design and Delivery of Long-Term Care Institutional Services

Upon admission to a nursing home or other long-term care setting, residents are limited in the extent to which they can make choices with respect to routine aspects of their lives such as diet and recreational activities. Major decisions about routine aspects of physical and emotional maintenance are made by administrative and direct care staff in the nursing home. For minority aged, the possibility of inconsistencies between self-perceived needs and needs as determined by long-term care staff is great, especially in facilities where ethnic and racial minority groups represent a small proportion of the resident body.

In meeting the psychosocial needs of minority aged in long-term care, it would seem important to consider their culturally accustomed patterns of eating, socializing and living in general. In other words, to program for cultural congruence or consistency.

Operationalizing the concept of cultural congruence is difficult. Recent research in this area holds promise for developing quality of care measures which consider sociocultural factors. Based on her studies of child welfare services to racial and ethnic minority children, including those in congregate care facilities, Jenkins has developed a conceptual and operational framework for assessing the extent to which commitment to ethnic factors is reflected in program design and implementation.[31]

A service delivery system's commitment to ethnic factors in meeting the needs of racial and ethnic minority clients can be assessed along three major dimensions, (1) attention to ethnic factors in program content, (2) matching versus mixing of staff and clientele on the basis of race or ethnicity, and (3) extent of ethnic minority input at the policy-making level.

Specific aspects of service design, staffing and decision-making have been identified by Jenkins as indicators of the degree of attention to ethnic concerns. Programming for cultural congruence could be determined by (1) use of ethnic foods on a routine basis, (2) use of culturally familiar music, art, dance, and recreational activities, (3) celebration of holidays important to minority clients, and (4) teaching staff about the importance of attention to cultural consistency in planning programs within the service system.

Matching versus mixing of clients and staff on the basis of ethnicity could be observed by ascertaining the racial or ethnic composition of staff vis-à-vis the resident population. In particular, how represented are ethnic or racial minority persons on the staff both at the administrative and direct care levels. How involved are minority staff members in designing and planning programs. Minority input at the policy and decision-making level could be determined by the race or ethnicity of the administrator and ethnic composition of the policy-making board.

Administrator Attitudes

Using this framework, Morrison interviewed nursing home administrators and 93 black aged residents about programming practices and attitudes regarding the importance of cultural congruence in programming and ethnic matching.

Because the study sample is small and limited to voluntary nursing homes in a specific locale (New York City), the findings should be viewed as illustrative of issues, rather than definitive.

Both administrator and resident attitudes were found to be related to a number of interdependent variables including ethnic and racial composition of the resident body, auspices of the nursing home, and ethnicity of the administrator.

Nursing homes built under the auspices of a black church or organization were most likely to program for cultural congruence. Their administrators were more likely to value ethnic or racial matching of staff and residents and to feel that the administrator should be of the same ethnic background as the majority of the residents. They were also more in favor of minority representation on the policy-making board as necessary to meeting the needs of minority residents. White administrators in homes serving a small percentage of black aged were less committed to cultural congruence as it pertains to aged blacks and indicated that the costs of meeting the specialized dietary and activity preferences of aged blacks would be too great given their small numbers in the resident population. Although white administrators favored hiring black staff "at all levels," they did not feel that ethnic or racial matching of the administrator or the policy-making board vis-à-vis the resident population was necessary to meet the needs of minority aged in long-term care.[32]

Administrators were asked if they supported the establishment of separate ethnic nursing homes designed and operated by blacks to care for their own aged. Black administrators were in favor of this and white administrators were not. Ironically, two of the white administrators were in nursing homes established by particular religious or ethnic groups to serve their own aged, although they currently have non-sectarian admission policies.

Each of the administrator's attitudes tended to match current programming practices. It is difficult to determine whether attitudes flow from practices or are shaped by them. Clearly the racial or ethnic composition of the resident population is a critical factor.

FMA found similar results and summed up the situation this way:

> . . .approximately 25% of the long-term care administrators interviewed by FMA failed to recognize the significance of psychosocial factors in the delivery of good care to racial/ethnic minority residents. Interestingly, these administrators were found in facilities with the lowest concentration of minority residents which may, in part, account for this attitude and low order of priority assigned to special (psychosocial) needs of cohort groups.[33]

Residents Attitudes

Attitudes of black aged residents were found to also relate to whether or not the residents were in a predominantly non-white or white facility—especially on issues of ethnic matching at the staff and decision-making levels.

Taken as a whole, black residents placed the most importance on programming for cultural congruence. There was significant support for celebration of holidays (especially religious holidays), church services which allowed residents to worship in their accustomed manner, and the regular provision of ethnic (usually "soul") foods. No significant differences were found between residents in predominantly black and predominantly white facilities with respect to the desire for cultural familiarity in food and activities. Residents in predominantly white facilities, however, were aware of the influence of racial and ethnic composition of the resident population on programming decisions. Expressed desires for ethnically familiar foods and activities were frequently qualified by statements such as "I would like these things, but I know there are too few of us here for anything to change."

Black residents were less in favor of ethnic or racial matching of staff and residents. The strongest overall support was for involving black staff in the design of programs in the nursing home (58%), followed by employment of black staff at all levels in the nursing home (48%). Only 27% of the residents in the study sample felt it was important for the nursing home administrator to be black. This appears to be one area where black residents took a different position from black administrators.

Those black aged in predominantly black facilities were on the average more likely to feel that ethnic matching was important compared to those in predominantly white facilities. Feelings about ethnic matching are complex. Their complexity must be understood in a sociohistorical context for most minority aged, and perhaps especially so for aged blacks whose lifetime experiences of forced racial segregation were so profound. Some resident comments will serve to illustrate. Residents in favor of ethnic matching favored it for several reasons. The most frequently expressed view was that one's own people understand you better. As one 80-year-old woman said, "The interest in old people is what's really important. But I do feel that our people know each other better—we know each other's troubles."

Others favored hiring black staff because of a desire for fairness in providing employment opportunities. One resident stated, "Our people have as much right to work here as anyone else. Anyway, we have more black people in here so it makes sense." Finally, others emphasized ethnic matching as an expression of anger and distrust of whites. One old man said, "It is very important to have colored people on the staff. I don't believe in the white man. I don't want whites here. White people can take of their own."

Residents who disapproved of ethnic matching also did so for varied reasons. The most typical reason for opposition was the association of ethnic matching as a policy with enforced racial segregation. As one resident put it, "I believe the staff should be mixed. No segregation. One of the main problems in this world is segregation." A related sentiment was the expression of a universal humanistic perspective which transcended racial or ethnic boundaries. "It doesn't matter to me what color the staff are as long as they have feeling. I am not a race person. What matters to me is humanity." Finally for some black residents, the presence of white administrative and direct care personnel was associated with a perception of better quality service.

These findings suggest that black aged are not a homogeneous group with respect to attitudes or preferences. Although core agreement was observed on importance of cultural congruence in programming, considerable variability was found on issues of racial or ethnic matching. Even residents who favored the same outcome, did so for varied reasons. The lesson in this is that there will always be individual variations on dominant cultural themes. An appreciation of this fact will avoid slipping easily into a stereotypic response, either at the programming or individual level.

Minority aged residents in long-term care will need to be individualized, even when dominant cultural themes are recognized and appreciated. This will be best assured when practitioners follow the basic social work precepts of starting where the client is and understanding his needs in relation to where he has been.

Variations in attitudes were also observed between aged residents from different ethnic groups. Dobrof and Morrison undertook an AoA-funded study of cultural and familial determinants of institutional placement.[34] In this study 52 Hispanic (predominantly Puerto Rican) aged and 36 Chinese aged were asked to state their preferences for cultural congruence in nursing home services and ethnic matching. Their responses were compared to those of aged blacks in the Morrison study. Statistically significant differences were found between the three groups on every area measured in the Jenkins framework, except for one: routine provision of ethnic foods which was favored by the vast majority of all three groups. Findings appear in Table 1.

Black and Hispanic aged placed greater importance on celebration of ethnic holidays than Chinese aged. The same pattern was observed with respect to holding church services which allowed worship in the accustomed manner. Hispanic aged were most likely to feel that staff should be taught about their culture (over 90%), but only two-thirds of the black aged held this view as did half of the Chinese aged.

Table 1

Scale Items	Ethnicity of the Resident			Significance Chi Square
	Black (n=93)	Hispanic (n=52)	Chinese (n=36)	

Resident Responses to the Jenkins Ethnic Commitment Scale, by Ethnicity of the Resident (Percentage)

Cultural Content

Scale Items	Black (n=93)	Hispanic (n=52)	Chinese (n=36)	Chi Square
Celebrate holidays	90	84	56	.001
Church services	86	90	11	.001
Ethnic foods	77	88	89	n.s.
Music, art	77	90	68	.001
Staff taught ethnic culture	68	90	50	.001
Transportation to church of choice	68	80	0	.001
Mixing vs. Matching				
Ethnic staff used in program design	58	82	81	.001
Ethnic staff employed at all levels	48	96	92	.001
Ethnic administration preferred	27	82	75	.001
Decision-Making				
Ethnic representation on the Board	71	84	22	.001
Supports separate ethnic nursing homes	50	88	100	.001

On issues of ethnic matching at the policy-making and direct care staff levels, Hispanics took the overall strongest position, followed by Chinese aged and then by blacks. Preference for an administrator from the same ethnic group showed the greatest variability across the three groups. Such a preference was expressed by 82% of the Hispanic aged, 75% of the Chinese aged and only 27% of the black aged. While black aged were split 50-50 on support for the establishment of separate ethnic nursing homes, 88% of the Hispanics and 100% of the Chinese supported the establishment of such facilities.

It is clear that generalizations about all "ethnic or minority" aged based on experiences with one group are risky, at best. In interpreting these findings, language issues may take on some importance. For non-English predominant groups such as Hispanic and Chinese aged, ethnic matching tyically means linguistic matching. Under these conditions residents are more likely to feel that their needs can be adequately communicated, as well as understood.

The research findings presented in this chapter should be considered illustrative of issues to be considered in the plan and operation of long-term care services to aged persons from ethnic minority groups. Much more empirical evidence is needed on provider and consumer attitudes. Most importantly, quality of care measures need to be developed which assess service quality along psychosocial and cultural dimensions, as well as biomedical ones. There are, however, some suggested guidelines for practitioners in long-term care settings which can be derived from the available data.

Suggested Guidelines for Practice

1. Providers of institutional long-term care need to do more outreach and information-giving in minority communities. Black churches, black social organizations and informal meetings held in schools or other available facilities can serve as channels for dissemination of information about services, application procedures, admission criteria and what families need to consider in making a placement decision. Social workers from referring hospitals and nursing homes are a natural to conduct such orientation meetings.

2. Hospital personnel, who now play a major role in referring minority aged to long-term care facilities, must be trained to provide minority families with the same range of information and options available to other families struggling with care-taking issues. No a priori assumptions should be made about a non-white family's receptivity to the nursing home as a viable option. Both the needs of the aged relative and other family members need to be realistically assessed in light of existing material, social and emotional resources. Institutional long-term care should be presented as one of several options to be considered.

3. In making referrals to nursing homes every effort should be made to match the aged persons needs with existing resources. Sociocultural, as well as biomedical, factors need to be considered in making this determination. Minority aged and their families should be openly asked about preferences for specific patterns of care, and where feasible, these preferences should be respected in making referrals.

4. Intermediate and skilled nursing facilities are needed in minority communities. Location has been shown to be an important factor in service utilization by minority aged. Minority group churches and business organizations might be approached to consider sponsorship of a nursing home based in their respective communities. Technical assistance in both the fiscal and operational management of the facility will be needed, as well as adequate funding to assure high quality services and personnel.

5. In designing programs in nursing homes and other long-term care facilities, cultural congruence vis-à-vis the resident population is critical. This tends to be especially important where ethnic minority aged represent a small percentage of the resident population. Facility administrators and staff must see the value of such programming for resident well-being, otherwise no commitment of time and resources will be made given real financial constraints in operating the facility. Social work staff can play a key role in sensitizing administrative personnel to the importance of considering quality of care in sociocultural terms. This role for social workers, of course, will depend on the extent to which they have been adequately trained to appreciate the importance of ethnic factors in service delivery. Whenever dominant cultural patterns are considered in designing menus or activities, staff should not forget that each resident is an individual.

6. In-service staff training will be needed to stress the importance of considering cultural factors in the design and delivery of services. Although consciousness-raising and attitudinal issues are important training areas, staff will be helped considerably by concrete suggestions on how to build in cultural components. Persons from the different ethnic groups who have knowledge of food preferences and social activities can be invited to do such training. Concrete suggestions around preparation of ethnic foods, use of culturally familiar handicrafts, music and other folklore can be made. Technical expertise in such areas can be sought from national and local minority aging organizations such as the National Caucus on the Black Aged and the National Organization of Hispanic Elderly. FMA noted in their report that The Bureau of Indian Affairs has given this type of assistance in programming for American Indian aged. When minority aged residents are well enough, they might be encouraged to share their expertise in the preparation of ethnic foods or handicrafts with other residents as part of group activities in the home. Staff can also learn from these activities of "cultural exchange."

7. Wherever minority aged are served, minority staff should be represented on the facility's administrative and direct care staff. Language

barriers to the effective delivery of services in institutional settings require that bilingual staff be used whenever possible. At the same time, English-speaking staff can be encouraged to learn languages represented among the resident population served. Special incentives through financial bonuses or special recognition awards could be given for undertaking additional study. The same could apply to taking courses which increase understanding of the cultural patterns of groups served.

8. Long-term care facilities should seek to maximize the involvement of family members and interested persons from the ethnic community in the resident's plan of care. Families and volunteers from the ethnic community can assist in planning social and recreation activities which will increase the probability of cultural congruence in programming.

9. Finally, quality assurance measures need to be developed and implemented which consider sociocultural dimensions, as well as biomedical ones. If one accepts the validity of caring for an institutionalized older person as a whole person, the plan of care must reflect attention to psychosocial needs as well as medical needs. Aged persons from ethnic and racial minority groups who are residents of long-term care facilities may require special assurances in this regard.

REFERENCES

1. Three such studies cited extensively in this chapter are: Eribes, Richard A., and Bradley-Rawls, Martha. "The Underutilization of Nursing Homes by Mexican-American Elderly in the Southwest," *The Gerontologist* 18(4), 1978, pp. 363-371. Forward Management Associates, Inc. *Final Report on the Study of the Special Needs of Racial/Ethnic Minorities and Provider Attitudes in Long Term Care Facilities-Educational Implications.* Contract No. HRA 230-76-0174, January 31, 1977; and Morrison, Barbara Jones, *Black Aged in Nursing Homes: An Application of the Shared Function Thesis.* Doctoral Dissertation, Columbia University. 1979.

2. Brody, Elaine & Sparks, Geraldine "Institutionalization of the Aged: A Family Crisis." *Family Process,* 5 (1), 1966, pp. 76-90, Zappolo, Aurora. *Characteristics, Social Contacts and Activities of Nursing Home Residents, United States, 1973-74* National Nursing Home Survey. Washington, D.C. DHEW, National Center for Health Statistics, Publication No. HRA 77-1778.

3. United States Department of Health and Human Services. *Characteristics of the Black Elderly.* DHEW Publication No. (OHDS) 80-20057, 1980.

4. *Ibid.,* p. 17.

5. Dowd, James J. & Bengston, Vern L. "Aging in Minority Populations." *Journal of Gerontology* 33 (3), 1978, pp. 427-436.

6. Cantor, Marjorie, "Health and the Inner City Elderly." Paper presented at the 27th Annual Meeting of the Gerontological Society, Portland Oregon, October, 1974.

7. Dowd & Bengston, *op cit.,* p. 431.

8. Eribes & Bradley-Rawls, *op. cit.,* p. 367.

9. USDHHS, Characteristics of the Black Elderly, *op. cit.,* p.16.

10. Rubenstein, Daniel I. "An Examination of Social Participation Found Among a National Sample of Black and White Elderly," *Aging and Human Development,* 2 (1971), pp. 172-173.

11. Cantor, Marjorie. "The Elderly in the Inner City: Some Implications of the Effects of Culture on Life Styles," (Paper presented at the Institute on Gerontology and Graduate Education for Social Work, New York City, Fordham University at Lincoln Center, March 20 1973), pp. 4-5.

12. Cantor, Marjorie. "The Elderly in the Inner City: Some Implications of the Effects of Culture on Life Styles," *op. cit.* Jackson, Jacquelyne. "Sex and Social Class Variations in Black Aged Parent-Adult-Child Relationships." *Aging and Human Development.* 2(2), 1971, pp. 96-107.

13. American Public Health Association. *Minority Health Chartbook.* Washington, D.C., U.S. Government Printing Office, 1974, p. 81.

14. Forward Management Associates, *op. cit.*

15. *Ibid.,* p. II-6.

16. Morrison, Barbara Jones. *Op. cit.,* p. 114.

17. Forward Management Associates, *op.cit.,* p. II-21.

18. Downing, Ruppert A. & Copeland, Elaine J. "Services for the Black Elderly: National or Local Problems?" *Journal of Gerontological Social Work,* 2 (4), 1980, p. 298.

19. Eribes & Bradley-Rawls, *op. cit.,* p. 366.

20. Forward Management Associates, *op. cit.,* p. II-8.

21. *Ibid.,* II-5.

22. Eribes & Bradley-Rawls, *op. cit.,* p. 366.

23. Forward Management Associates, *op. cit.,* p. II—6.

24. *Ibid.,* pp. II-6-II-7

25. *Ibid.,* p. II-7.

26. *Ibid.*

27. Eribes & Bradley-Rawls, *op.cit.,* p. 368.

28. *Ibid.*

29. Forward Management Associates, *op. cit.,* p. III-5.

30. Forward Management Associates, *op. cit.,* p. II-6.

31. Jenkins, Shirley. *The Ethnic Dilemma in Social Services,* New York: The Free Press, 1981. See Chapter 3: "The Ethnic Agency Defined," pp. 43-74.

32. Morrison, Barbara. *op. cit.,* pp. 138-142.

33. Forward Management Associates, *op. cit.,* p. III-3.

34. Dobrof, Rose & Morrison, Barbara. "Path to the Institution: SocioCultural, Familial and Organizational Factors," Brookdale Center on Aging of Hunter College (CUNY), AoA Grant No.90-A-1668/01, 1980.

Part III

PERSPECTIVES FROM
THE WORLD OF PRACTICE

Chapter 8

COMMUNITY CARE FOR THE AGED:
THE NATURAL SUPPORTS PROGRAM

Anna H. Zimmer

The increasing concern about planning for long-term care of the aged in the community has led to the "rediscovery" of their natural supports— family, friends and neighbors. Although the aged have traditionally been cared for by this informal network, until the mid 1970s few social services were designed to meet their needs. It was not until the research studies of Cantor[1] and Shanas[2] dispelled the myth of the abandoned aged that we began to systematically examine the nature and extent of care provided by the natural supports. In 1977, Elaine Brody[3] stated . . . "The responsible behavior of families towards older people has been so thoroughly documented that it is no longer an issue in gerontological research." As noted in the report of the General Accounting Office,[4] the overall estimate is that about 80% of all services received by impaired older persons are provided informally by kinsmen and friends.

This description of an innovative service for the natural supports of the aged in the community is based upon the pioneer work of the Community Service Society[5] Natural Supports Program. Building upon extensive experience in serving the aged through its Older Person Service, CSS in 1976 initiated the NSP. During the period 1976-1981 two different service modalities were implemented by the program. The first, task-centered social casework with caregiving families; the second, the development of community based support groups[6] for family, friends and neighbors of the disabled elderly.

The main thrust of both approaches has been to strengthen and enhance the care giving capacity of the natural supports, rather than act as a sub-

This article is adapted from a presentation "Fostering Natural Support Systems, Innovations and Trends" at the 109th Annual Forum of the National Conference on Social Welfare, April 27 1982, Boston, MA.

149

stitute for their efforts. From the onset, the possibility of "overloading" the informal network or even considering a return to filial responsibility was recognized as a danger to be avoided.

The majority of caregivers who participated in the program were employed daughters caring for a frail older parent. The largest group were aged 50-59 years although a high proportion were themselves over 65 years of age. The second most significant group of caregivers were spouses and, thirdly, siblings. The older person being cared for was most often widowed, female and over 75 years of age. Disabilities were of long standing, chronic in nature and the recipient of care generally required a high level of attention. The help needed included shopping, bathing, feeding and assistance related to a significant memory loss. All caregivers reported that they provided emotional support to the care recipient and, furthermore, this was one of the hardest caregiving tasks to perform.

Individual Services to Families

The family interview, with all available caregivers and the older person, was used for the initial assessment. During this interview the family participated in determining the amount of continuing care to be provided by the family members and helped in planning the service design. A letter of agreement formalized the outcome of the family meeting, the type and duration of service provided by the family and by the agency and allowed for periodic review and modification. Casework service was available for both the caregiver and for the older person as requested and was delivered in home visits or office interviews.[7] Services to families included home care, respite for the caregivers, counselling, escort service and assistance in systems negotiations and advocacy directed toward securing entitlements for the older person. The caseworker was called upon to adapt services to the individual famly pattern, often in a more flexible fashion than the system provided i.e., home care in less than 4 hour units or adjusted to a working daughter's schedule. Families responded positively to the availability of the service and noted especially that this was the first time that their role and their needs were recognized, e.g., evening and weekend hours for casework interviews were scheduled if the family members were working during the daytime. The following is an example of a typical situation encountered by a middle-aged daughter caring for a disabled mother.

Mr. and Mrs. A., a childless couple, had looked forward to their retirement as a chance to enjoy their time together. Instead, Mrs. A. become overly concerned about her 90-year-old mother, Mrs. G., who had been living with them for 7 years. She now required help with dressing, toileting and meal preparation. Her confusion about time and place necessitated almost full time supervision. Mrs. A., in adjusting to her own retirement and the responsibility for her mother, lost weight, was anxious and conflicted about her loyalties to her mother and husband. At the family meeting Mrs. A. was seeking some respite while Mr. A.'s request was, "tell her what's enough to do for her mother." Regular counselling for Mrs. A. was provided along with funds for a twice-a-week companion aide for Mrs. G. Mrs. A. worked through some of her guilt and fears and reset her priorities. Thus, when her mother deteriorated further, she was able to apply for public home care entitlements for her. Currently, a home attendant comes 5 mornings a week and Natural Supports Program provides a monthly allowance which the A's use for evening respite. Mr. A. now fully retired, is sharing part of the care of his mother-in-law. They enjoy their evenings out together, are each involved in some adult education and although Mrs. A. is still "an only child caring for mother" she seems to have found some balance in her roles, as retired person, wife and daughter.

Group Services

The second service modality was the development of community-based support groups. The notion of a continuum of informal social supports developed by Gerald Caplan[8] has been very valuable in the development of groups for caregivers.

Caplan sees the continuum consisting of kin, friends and neighbors, non-professional community persons, religious denominations, fraternal orders, mutual assistance, and self-help groups. Caplan has discovered in a modern idiom, what Petr Kropotkin noted earlier, "And the need of mutual aid and support which had lately taken refuge in the narrow circle of the family or the slum neighbors, in the village or the secret union of workers, reasserts itself again, even in our modern society . . ."[9]

A group work practice framework must accept the simultaneous generalized nature of material, cognitive-emotive and instrumental resources supplied by the informal social support system.

Community-based group services were developed for family, friends and neighbors of the aged in collaboration with a variety of local agencies or groups i.e., an inter-Agency Council on Aging, a senior center, religious or fraternal organizations. The meetings were of two types—community wide educational meetings, to which caregivers were invited via flyers and general publicity, or small informal discussion groups, generally hosted by one specific service agency which invited targeted "known" caregivers to attend. The group meetings were offered as a means by which those caring for an older person might obtain information and help.[10]

The focus of caregiver groups was to supplement and reinforce efforts of kin and friends particularly when they were unable to maintain their assistance because of conflicting pressures in the kinship network, changes in the elderly person's health status and fluctuations in the caregiver's physical and emotional capacity to provide help. The small group's mutual aid processes had the potential to support the self-help efforts of kin and friends. Recognizing the strength in caregivers, the group development was continued for small ongoing peer-support groups that could move towards self-help. Enabling services were provided by CSS or the local sponsors in the form of a group facilitator, counselling, meeting space, home care for the older person to allow caregiver meeting attendance and transportation as requested.

Caregivers attending groups were seeking information (especially about entitlements for the older person) skills training and peer support. A number of caregivers also needed individual service to address crisis problems before they could utilize group services. Any comprehensive caregiver program should therefore provide for this as an enabling service.

The CSS experience suggests that ongoing groups move through various stages of development. The first stage is one of meeting concrete service needs (education and skills training). The second is the development of peer support and the third is an advocacy or social action stage.[11] Parallel to this progression through the three phases was a development towards self-help, which was consciously encouraged by the staff facilitators. The following example illustrates both these trends during the life of one group[12]

Group A consisted of 6-8 women in their late fifties and sixties, black, white and Hispanic, who were caring for a parent, relative or spouse.

A series of six community-wide meetings were planned entitled "Caring for Older Relatives." Outreach for the meeting consisted of flyers and publicity to the service agencies. As a result of the first few topical informational meetings, several women indicated that they would like to continue meeting on an ongoing basis. A professional social worker facilitated the first meeting which was held at a community senior center. At the outset she stated that she would be available for four meetings after which the participants might want to continue alone on a self-help basis with her assistance as a resource person. After the initial introductions the facilitator explained that the group was convened in response to members' needs, "this is your group" and asked the participants how they wanted to use the sessions. Two members immediately responded by requesting information about entitlements for the aged so that they "might better help" their friends. The facilitator promised that in addition to providing information, she would teach the participants how they could gather their own information and stressed how they might help each other by pooling what knowledge they each possessed.

The facilitator, throughout, encouraged participants to offer suggestions to each other and asked one member to gather information about services to share with the group at its next meeting. The next three meetings followed much the same format with the facilitator underscoring and encouraging mutual aid between members.

At the fourth and final meeting, the leader recognized the group's interest in continued meetings, and facilitated discussion of time, place and frequency. One member volunteered her home as a meeting site. Then the leader asked whether the group wanted to be open or closed. The group chose open membership at which point the leader requested permission to refer appropriate caregivers. As another way of transferring leadership, the facilitator gave resource booklets to the group for future distribution to members. She clarified her role in relation to the group after this session, reminding the members that she would no longer be meeting with them regularly but that she would be available to help them with any concerns as needed. She has since maintained a regular phone contact with one member, providing technical assistance around resource information and group technique. Although the professional facilitator was invited to attend whenever she could she chose to remain physically distant from the group and only once returned since this time.

The group met monthly over a two year period providing each of its members with peer support and mutual aid, and individual members became involved in publicizing the group and stressing the needs of caregivers, taking an active part in public testimony.

The group was unwilling to sever completely the contact with the professional network. This contact was seen as a lifeline and support if professional intervention was needed and represented professional acknowledgment of the caregiving effort.

The skills utilized by social workers in the two service modalities described have long been part of the social workers' expertise. However the needs and potential of caregivers as they face increasing demands call for innovative responses from the formal network and an adaptation of the social workers' role from group leader to that of enabler and facilitator. The formal services described here can enhance the caregivers' role and enable them to continue with less stress. Strengthening not substitution is the underlying guideline and when this occurs the "right" balance between the formal and the informal caregiving systems is attained.

REFERENCES

1. Cantor, Marjorie H. Life Space and the Social Support System of the Inner City Elderly of New York City. Gerontologist 15: pp. 23-27.

2. Shanas, Ethel. The Family as a Social Support System in Old Age. Presented at the Symposium on Natural Support Systems for the Elderly, 30th Annual Meeting of the Gerontological Society, San Francisco, 1980.

3. Brody, Elaine. Care of the Elderly, New York, 1977, p. 91.

4. U.S. General Accounting Office, The Well Being of Older People in Cleveland, Ohio, 1977. U.S. Government Printing Office.

5. The Community Service Society of New York is one of the oldest private non-profit, non-sectarian social agencies in the U.S.

6. The Community Service Society Natural Supports Community Group Development was funded in part by grant #02AM-4802 from the Model Projects, Administration on Aging, Department of HHS.

7. For a more detailed description of program design see; Gross-Andrew, Susannah and Zimmer, Anna H. "Incentives to Families Caring for Disabled Elderly: Research and Demonstration Project to Strengthen the Natural Support System." Paper presented at the 30th Annual Scientific Meeting, San Francisco, November 20 1977 and published in *Journal of Gerontological Social Work*, Vol. 1, no. 2, Winter, 1979. P. 119.

8. Caplan, Gerald. *Support Systems and Community Mental Health,* New York: Behavioral Publications, 1974.

9. Kropotkin, Petr. *Mutual Aid: A Factor of Evolution,* Boston: Extending Horizon Books, 1902, p. 292. Republished, undated.

10. Hudis, Iris, Zimmer, Anna H., Sainer, Janet S. & Fulchon, Chinita. "A Group Program for Families of the Aging: A Service Strategy for Strengthening Natural Supports."

Paper presented at the 30th Annual Scientific Meeting, Gerontological Society, San Francisco, Nov. 20 1977. Published as "Strengthening Natural Supports: A Group Program for Families of the Aging" in M. Teicher, D. Thursz, and J. Vigilante (Eds.) *Social Service Delivery Systems: An International Annual,* Vol. 4; Reaching the Aged: Social Services in Forty-Four Countries, pp. 53-64. Beverly Hills; Sage Publications, 1979.

11. Zimmer, Anna H. and Hudis, Iris E. "Education for Caregivers of the Aged: A Development View," Paper presented at the 33rd Annual Scientific Meeting, Gerontological Society, San Diego, California, November 23, 1980.

12. Mellor, Joanna, Rzetelny, Harriet & Hudis, Iris. "Self-Help Groups for Caregivers of the Aged." Paper presented at the 1st Annual Symposium, "Social Work with Groups," Cleveland, Ohio, December 1, 1979.

Chapter 9

ADULT DAY CARE:
EXPANDING OPTIONS FOR SERVICE

Rose Goldstein

What is missing in the lives of many of our elderly, who are struggling to maintain a level of independence, control and decision-making, is the availability of community services that respond to individual needs and offer the older person the freedom of choice. In trying to help these clients decide on an effective plan, the social worker is confronted by meager options of community programs and must creatively ferret out those fragmented services that are available. The choice of day care as a means of providing services to the frail and disabled elderly in the community has been limited to scattered demonstration programs throughout the country.

Day care as a concept of service did not grow out of society's commitment to older people or in recognition of their needs. With the advent of Medicare and Medicaid, program planning for the elderly moved in the direction of institutionalization. When institutions were no longer cost-effective and the public became aware that old people are a heterogeneous group with many different problems and needs, experimenting with an increasing variety of services to the elderly began. One of these services was day care.[1]

Emerging from a need to explore alternatives to institutionalization and contain costs, day care program development, adequate funding, standards and regulations have been slow to develop and erratic in meeting peoples needs. Some demonstration programs now in progress are Medicaid funded while others creatively tap local, state, and federal monies to put together a reimbursement package.

Day care for geriatric patients with medical-nursing components is not well developed in the United States. Where there are no day care services, aged people faced with physical and mental decline have been forced to choose institutionalization or community isolation. Adult day

157

care in the United States is primarily associated with psychiatric patients, as was the initial experience in the United Kingdom.[2]

In researching the community approach to geriatric health care, McCuan and Levenson point out that historically, the day treatment center has roots in the European day hospital movement which was originally applied to the geriatric mental patient. This concept has recently been expanded to include the physically-impaired and the chronically-ill aged.[3]

Although day care programs begin with the idea that they are alternatives to institutionalization, and for many aged, institutionalization has been delayed or permanently interrupted, day care can provide the option for a more meaningful community life.

There are marginally functioning aged in the community with different needs but with a common determination to remain independent: the isolated who will not reach out for services; the mentally impaired for whom there are few services; and the medically fragile who need continuous monitoring. Many are loners, some with history of depression, paranoia or schizoid personality, and many with moderate dementia. They often have a myriad of illnesses—cardiovascular disease, arthritis, hypertension, diabetes, post CVA, and visual impairment. The traditional community clubs for aged, senior centers and church groups, do not attract these frail and disabled clients and are not prepared to serve them. Many of these men and women are fearful of venturing out to make use of community resources. Because of their special needs, primarily medical and psychosocial monitoring and a more individual level of intervention, they are best helped in a small day care program that has nursing, social services, medical and rehabilitation services available.

Day Care in the Institution

Observations and case histories in this paper are based on experiences at the Day Care Program of the non-profit Jewish Home & Hospital for Aged, at Kingsbridge Center in the Bronx. Begun in 1974 and funded through Medicaid, the program has provided necessary services in a live-at-home approach. Housed in a multilevel geriatric complex, the Day Care Center also offers transportation, a hot lunch, recreational activities, and many ancillary medical services. This is a 5-day-a-week program serving 40 participants each day, with a total clientele of 80 members.

Elizabeth Gustafson points out that long-term care facilities in most states are already licensed by definition to provide day care, since day care is, from a regulatory point of view, a lesser service.[4]

Koff sees the institution as especially suited to provide the base for non-institutional service because of its competence, specialized staff, commitment for continuity of care and concern for the community. The institution can take two roles, one for supporting non-institutional services within its own setting and, secondly, the use of the setting's knowledge in the development of non-institutional service within the total community.[5] In addition to being housed in residential health care facilities, day care programs can be offered in non-institutional congregate settings which meet local regulations and older people's needs.

Generally day care centers primarily serve individuals who are limited physically and psychosocially, and are designed to maintain maximum functioning in the community. In addition to nursing and medical assessments day care participants need to be assessed by the social worker to identify the ego strengths and mastery that have helped them to remain in the community. At the Kingsbridge Day Care Center this information is incorporated into a care plan that is shared with the individual's private physician, through a close liaison with a day care nurse and a social worker. The individual's physician bears the primary responsibility for the participant's medical needs. This arrangement, when built into a day care program, can provide the client with overall medical monitoring, appropriate referrals to ancillary medical services and necessary follow up, particularly in the area of medications.

The day care client who is temporarily unable to attend the program or requires hospitalization, benefits from a close contact and monitoring by the day care social worker and the day care nurse until ready to return to the program. In the frequent incidents of hip fractures or mild cardiovascular accidents, the goal would be to institutionalize the person for several weeks. The institution could provide rehabilitation therapy and help in preparing the client to return to the community at the highest level of function. Very often, when temporary institutionalization is indicated, it is important for the social worker to arrange the placement.

Referral and Intake

The day care client may be referred to the program by local community agencies, hospitals, departments of social services, community physicians, Visiting Nurse Service, local departments of aging, and families. Because the day care client may be emotionally or medically unstable, there is often a great deal of initial resistance to entering the program. Resistance may be due to fears of socialization or change in one's daily routine, depression, physical illness or an inability to understand the day care program. The social worker has to convince the person to give the program a trial period. Older people must experience a service in order to fully comprehend what the service has to offer.

Intake in a day care program should begin with an in-depth interview with the social worker, exploring the client's past and current lifestyles, level of function and community supports. Despite mental and physical impairments, clients often need encouragement to set realistic goals in which they can participate. If a family member makes the referral and the social worker determines that the family member is involved in the daily life of the applicant, the family should participate in the setting of the goals. Developing a partnership between the applicant and day care, around the older person's goals and expectations for services and supports is the beginning step in reaching for mastery and reinforcing ego strengths. "What can day care do to help to make your life better in the community?" This is the magic question that is asked and reasked and rephrased for each person's understanding. An example of the process is the following case.

> Mrs. I., a 72-year-old widow, shared a 2½-room apartment with a 35-year-old bachelor son, in a deteriorated neighborhood. She was referred by a local senior center which could not manage her disturbed behavior. Diagnosed Ambulatory Schizophrenic, Mrs. I. reluctantly came for several initial interviews. First she wanted help with getting her apartment painted, then someone to talk to and some days her arthritis pain "nearly killed her." With a sensitive one-to-one approach by the social worker, and with lots of distance for her to move away when necessary, she entered the program. Her lifetime pattern of marginal relatedness and her ambivalence about attending day care caused havoc in transportation scheduling. She would miss the driver, wait on the wrong corner or on the wrong day. Mrs. I. met with the social worker for 15 minutes each day she came to day care. This helped reduce her anxiety and ultimately to separate her from her son. When her son decided to move out and marry, the social worker supported her through a very agitated depression, accompanied her to the wedding, helped her to relocate to a more appropriate apartment, and continued to follow her in day care. A care plan around her ambivalence and changing expectations was worked out and continuously reassessed.

Comprehensive Services

A day care program can offer a broad spectrum of professional services encompassing the informal social supports that the community may no longer provide. During the 5 or 6 compact hours that the person is in day care, the services may range from rehabilitation to nursing and social services and include recreation, dietary, socializing, education, personal care, exercise, transportation, and other therapeutic services that help maintain function and independence. However, for day care to be an effective program, it cannot be an 8A.M.-2P.M. or a 9A.M.-3P.M. day for the clients, social worker or the nurse. A comprehensive care plan must include assistance for the participants in managing their lives during the hours and days when day care is not open.

The social worker's clinical intervention draws on the client's past mastery. The social worker must practice with the awareness that old people continue to learn, and "solving" a person's problems interferes with learning. The exercise of responsibility through participation in the solving of one's daily problems is often considered as indicative of continued growth, and significantly related to life satisfaction in the later years.[6]

No matter what the task, there are steps in the helping process that call on the client's capacity for some self-direction and for maintaining a sense of control, i.e., if the social worker assesses the client's need for household help to continue functioning in the community, step 1 is helping the client to obtain the service, and step 2 is teaching the client how to effectively supervise the helper, as in the case of Mrs. S.:

> An 83-year-old widow, Mrs. S. lived alone in a 3rd floor walkup. She managed marginally but independently despite many medical problems. Attended day care 3 days-a-week. Within a 5-month period, she lost a son, a granddaughter committed suicide, and she sustained a hip fracture from a fall. A social worker worked with a community doctor and Department of Social Services to obtain 24-hour home attendant during the critical weeks following return from hospital. Because services in the community were fragmented and slow in responding, this was time-consuming task that was stressful and frustrating to the worker. When help became available, a social worker counselled Mrs. S. to prevent her from becoming totally dependent on the home health attendant. Mrs. S. became comfortable with directing the attendant and did not have to give up control of how she wanted things done in her apartment.

When able to use a walker, Mrs. S. was assisted in locating another apartment in an elevated building. Through worker's intervention (home visits and telephone), Mrs. S. supervised her own packing and moving, despite recurring depression. She returned to day care after 3 months. Family stopped pressuring Mrs. S. to enter a nursing home, following social worker's contacts and meetings with family.

From whatever sources funding is obtained, day care reimbursement is only for the number of hours the participant is in the program. Client centered service is the critical component in a day care program, despite the fact that community follow up by the social worker is often squeezed into an already pressured and demanding day.

As part of the team approach, the Kingsbridge Day Care Program has developed a Home Health Team composed of the nurse, social worker, and occupational therapist. To assist the team in the total assessment of the individual's ability to function safely and effectively in the community, the team makes home visits to new members and regularly scheduled visits to people in the program. Questions considered are: Does the person need safety appliances in the bathroom; are the locks and windows secure; are there unused and unnecessary medications; where are they kept; is there appropriate food in the refrigerator; is there sufficient lighting; does the client need a referral for homemaking services.

Since memory impairment in the marginally-functioning older person is exacerbated by anxiety over the misplacement of keys and handbags in the person's apartment, the team addresses this problem and attempts to create a functional solution at the time of the visit. The removal of a slippery scatter rug that is a hazard to a person with impaired vision or poor ambulation, but has been on that floor for 25 years, is sensitively handled. Simple education for reading dates on food containers taught in the day care program is reinforced during the home visit.

The overall objective of day care is to stabilize the aged person's functional deficits and to enable him or her to maintain as much independent functioning as possible. In their research, McCuan and Levenson found that the key to successful service outcome is the ability to prevent the individual from slipping below the realistic level of independence, and wherever possible help the person fulfill his potential for independent living.[7]

To do this, the social worker needs a 3-pronged approach: (1) mobilize client's strengths so client can effectively use day care's concrete services to maintain a meaningful life in the community, (2) mobilize client's community network of supports, systems and medical care, (3) follow participant through community crises, illness, hospitalization, loss and interruption of entitlements. This was effectively done in the case of Mrs. P.

> When Mrs. P., a 78-year-old paranoid woman, appeared to function in day care but was causing havoc in the community, the social worker contacted and worked with the maintenance man in Mrs. P.'s building, so that he would be available during periods of crisis. This plan maintained Mrs. P.'s stability for 3 months. It had to be revised by the social worker, when the client decided the maintenance man was "one of them." The social worker then found a neighbor Mrs. P. had begun to trust. The social worker helped neighbor to understand Mrs. P.'s paranoid behavior and how to respond to Mrs. P. during paranoid episodes.

Isolation, often associated with illness in the aged, can be interrupted by the low-keyed socialization that a day care program can offer. Isolation, when permitted to continue, is often a deterrent to fostering and maintaining a maximum state of well-being.[8] Since low-keyed socialization is also therapeutic, it should characterize the day care milieu. This will subsequently help the isolate reenter a world of peer relationships.

Mr. O., a 75-year-old widower, who lived alone is an example of the positive effects of interrupting isolation.

> Mr. O. had not been out of his apartment for three years following two strokes which left his gait poor and unsteady. He was depressed, expressed fears of socialization and took no role in the management of his household. A home health attendant supervised his activities of daily living. "I talk to my TV," was his general comment. He was referred to day care by his doctor. The social worker, physical therapist and nurse made home visits to help him with his depression and teach him to negotiate one flight of stairs so he could meet the day care vehicle. After one month, Mr. O. was able to meet the day care car and attend three days a week. He met with the social worker, was enrolled in the rehabilitation program, and was getting about with the use of a walker. His general health improved and his depression lifted. He started socializing and became an active participant in group programs.

To remain independent in the community, most day care clients need the same things—acceptance, a structured environment that is responsive to their needs, and an opportunity to be listened to. Group process provides a basis for answering some of these needs.[9] Small problem solving groups led by the social worker are an essential program component of a day care setting. These groups of 5 to 8 people may cover such areas as marriage, mothers of schizophrenic children, living alone, and coping in the community. Specialty or task-oriented groups led by social worker, nurse or activity worker deal with nutrition, poetry, health care, safety and encourage social interaction so critical to a lonely, depressed aged person.

Responding to the needs of the client sets the tone for informal and formal program planning. For many of the marginal day care clients, a small group experience is an opportunity to risk social involvement. The restoration of self-determination and self-esteem are often obtained through social workers encouragement and discussion of complaints.[10] A day care setting affords the older person the opportunity to argue, to complain and compete. The ambiance is one of acceptance. The social environment is non-threatening and has the built-in support of concrete services. The world of the frail elderly in a day care program is more structured and as a result, the clients are less anxious. The members know the parameters of their helping network. The anxiety, of whom will I turn to with a social, medical, or community problem is minimized.

Mutual Aid

Through meetings with the social worker, members may be encouraged to become involved with one another when away from the program, creating a service of mutual aid among participants and maintaining social contacts in the community, in a concerned and caring way. This is reminiscent of a more meaningful way of living. The informal helping network encourages day care members to call each other on weekends, or when they are ill, and keep in touch in the event they need help in the community. Many of the fragile members of day care programs can only stay in touch by telephone since they are fearful of going out and have difficulty ambulating.

In metropolitan cities, where many elderly live alone and where sometimes the older person is one of the few remaining members of an earlier ethnic community, and is an alien in the midst of newcomers, day care means exchanging a dreary, lonely, often cold apartment for 5 hours, one to five days a week, for a program that fulfills so many of the older person's medical, psychological and social needs.[11]

One very traumatic loss for today's elderly is the loss of the next door neighbor who, for a largely immigrant population, was the somebody on whose door they could knock for help in an emergency, for daily companionship, for a sharing of the joys and sorrows of living. A responsive day care staff and peer interaction can provide the socialization and human contact which so many find lacking in their isolated community lives. The personality who cannot cope with the daily stresses of living looks to day care for the supports that the next door neighbor or family can no longer provide, as in the case of Mrs. W.:

> Social worker received a frantic call from Mrs. W., an 82-year-old widow, living alone and attending day care 3 days per week. She is diabetic and has a heart condition. She said she had a terrible problem, tried to call her daughter who was not at home, and decided not to upset her son. Problem: Mrs. W.'s only white neighbor died during the night. Although she did not know how she could get along without her dependable neighbor, she knew that she would never consider entering an institution, a suggestion her children often made. Social worker calmed and reassured Mrs. W. and subsequently arranged a meeting with Mrs. W. and family, to make plans for a move to a more suitable apartment.

Family Relations

In our urban centers, day care often has a unique and positive effect on the relationship between the aged person who lives alone in one part of a city, and his/her children who live in another. Their communication is often by telephone and the substance of the conversation, as reported to workers, is the complaints that pass between them. The parent is angry, lonely and frightened. The adult child is caring, but pressured, burdened by his own problems and unable to meet his parents needs. "We dread calling mother because all she does is complain. I wish she would agree to go into the Institution," is often heard. In a day care program the older person often has someone to share his complaints with, and is no longer dependent on that telephone call for total emotional support and meaningful contacts. Problems are shared with social worker, nurse, secretary, and driver. These are the people who respond to the day-to-day medical and psychosocial needs of the day care members. As a result, conversation between parent and child is about day care, medical services, activities, and socialization. Since adult children are less pressured by their parents, they in turn reduce their pressure for institutionalization. The anxiety as to whether mother is eating or taking her medication is greatly reduced, because of the contacts with the day care social worker and the nurse.

Families of participants often reach out to the day care social worker for help with community services, problems in understanding the behavior of aged parents and support in coping with parents' sudden illness and depression. Most children experience difficulty in dealing with the stresses evoked by a dependent, frail parent. A change in the older person's health, the need for additional services or different services will bring the family member to the social worker. Where appropriate, the social worker and nurse meet jointly with family to discuss change in medical or social functioning and evaluate participants' ability to continue independent community living.

In response to a crisis, the social worker will meet with the family members(s) and the participant in a joint interview, to explore alternatives and choices to effectively handle the crisis. Adult children often express a desire to support their parents emotionally, but feel helpless in handling psychological problems.

In working with family member(s), it is important for the social worker to assess how the family communicates, how crises were handled in the past, and what social, emotional, and financial resources are available to the client.

With the social worker's support, through the back-up services of a day care program, more families are able to accept a role in the community care of their older relative.

In some smaller urban centers like the Levindale Day Care Program in Baltimore, where the elderly continue to live with their families, a day care program could relieve the families of the responsibility for caring for these people during the day and provide a socializing experience for the participants.[12] The program might prolong their living in the community or possibly preclude placement in an institution. This service is especially important for the mentally impaired elderly, as in the case of Mrs. A., age 88, who lives with an unmarried daughter.

> Although the other siblings are interested in institutionalization because of Mrs. A.'s severe memory loss and cardiac condition, the family is aware that the shock of placement and change would

further impair her limited functioning. Mrs. A.'s daughter brought her mother to day care asking for a two days a week program, so the daughter could have some relief from the care of her mother. Mrs. A. is a pleasant, good-natured woman who compensates for her memory loss by her friendliness, but needs to be constantly supervised or she will wander. She is given simple tasks in occupational therapy and connected to other mentally frail participants in a supervised group. Mrs. A.'s initial separation from her daughter was reflected in severe anxiety about the fear of being lost, and being abandoned. Daughter meets with social worker for support in working through her anxieties in caring for a mentally impaired parent, and the possibility that institutionalization may at some time be indicated.

Day Care Challenge

Day care is a challenge to the participants who attend the program and to the staff who provide the services. For the impaired and fragile clients, the challenge is mobilizing one's resources to be able to get to the day care center. For some it is an opportunity to maintain a level of independence and experience choice in day-to-day living. For others it means staying out of the institution. But for most elderly who attend day care, the challenge is to make life in the community more meaningful through a sense of belonging and identification with people who care.

For staff the challenge often is to creatively put together a funding package, to provide client-centered service, despite community obstacles and fragmented services, and to engage the marginal isolated elderly and help them effectively utilize day care services.

Many states are now in the process of writing legislation that will amend their public health laws and social services laws in relation to the development and regulation of Adult day care services.

The National Institute on Adult Day Care (NIAD), organized in 1979 as a unit of the National Council on the Aging, lists as one of its purposes to promote the concept of adult day care as a viable community based option for disabled older persons within the larger continuum of long-term care.

Since the country now has 25.5 million people aged 65 and over, perhaps the real challenge is to recognize the different needs of the aged and to provide viable options through services and programs so that the elderly may find answers to the needs of their own life situations.

REFERENCES

1. Gustafson, Elizabeth. "Day Care for The Elderly," *Gerontologist*, February, 1974, Volume 14, No. 1, p. 47.

2. Mason, W. Dean. "Elderly Day Care Service in the USA-A Viable Option," *Nursing Homes*, January/February, 1978, p. 6.

3. McCuan, E.R. and Levenson, J. "Geriatric Day Care: A Community Approach to Geriatric Health Care," *Journal of Gerontological Nursing*, July/August 1977, Volume 3, No. 4, p. 43.

4. Gustafson, E. *Op cit.*, p.47.

5. Koff, T. H. "Rationale for Services: Day Care, Allied Care and Coordination," *Gerontologist*, February, 1974, Volume 14, No. 1, p. 29.

6. Kurtz, John J. and Kyle, David G. "Life Satisfaction & The Exercise of Responsibility," *Social Work*, July, 1977, Volume 22, No. 4, p. 324.

7. McCuan, E.R. and Levenson J. *Op cit.*, p. 43.

8. Robins, E.G. "Therapeutic Day Care," Paper presented at the Gerontology Society 27th Annual Meeting, Portland, Ore., October 30, 1974.

9. Turbow, S. "Geriatric Group Day Care and its Effect on Independent Living," *Gerontologist*, December, 1975, Volume 15, No. 6, p. 509.

10. Cohen, M.G. "Alternatives to Institutional Care of Aged," *Social Casework*, October, 1973, Volume 54, No. 8, p. 451.

11. Rabinowitz, D. and Nielsen, L. *"Home Life: A Story of Old Age,"* New York: The Macmillan Company, 1971, p. 24.

12. Kostick, A. "Levindale Day Care Program," *Gerontologist*, Volume 14, No. 1, February, 1974, p. 31.

Chapter 10

COLLABORATION IN A HOSPITAL: THE CASE OF THE DYING WOMAN

Susan Rubenstein
Marilyn Wilson

In its broadest sense, collaboration depends on working together towards a common goal. Whether it be in science or the lively arts, collaboration requires an integrated approach to problem solving with shared responsibility and good feeling among the participants for its outcome. Unlike collaborators in the arts, however, who willingly merge their individual talents, temperaments and individualities for a final seamless effect, the participants in health settings frequently have difficulties even agreeing on a common goal. Perhaps this is because our concept of collaboration has traditionally emphasized only the professional activity in behalf of a patient's well-being. Today's increasing discovery that social and psychological factors influence illness forces us to embrace the patient and family as equal participants in the collaborative process. This is never more important than in those instances of conflict which not uncommonly arise between the physician's mandate to heal and the patient's right to self-determination. Persisting conflicts of this sort leave in their wake angry medical staffs, misunderstood patients and frustrated social workers who may be unsure of helpful interventions.

In no social work setting is the dilemma between mere existence and its ensuing quality more visible and harrowing for choice than in an acute care hospital. By virtue of multiple frailties the case of the sick elderly is even more magnified. Jonathan Swift wished someone, "May you live all the days of your life!"[1] "May you live" is wonderfully juxtaposed to "all the days of your life" to emphasize each phrase's singular importance and difference before the total is melded into a new, fuller concept. So the physician's likely emphasis on "May you live" is extended to the elderly patient's immediacies concerning "all the days of

169

(my) life" to become at times a more wholesome concession and conclusion to patient care.

Out of a dual commitment to the best objectives of physician and patient grow the many social work interventions generally called collaborative work. The theme of existence and its quality becomes the double dimension or the encirclement of the social worker, defining his function and determining his unique contribution. This results in the social worker's alertness to the physician's mandate to preserve life—no mean possession—and the validity of the patient's multiple concerns with long-standing values attending his individual life. The trick resides in the collaborative techniques needed to bring both goals to a conclusion which is more or less acceptable to both physician and patient. The social work effort hopefully will never leave a patient perceived as "obstructive" nor a physician as "arbitrary." Different but equal values and goals emerge to survive for individually or mutually determined decisions. Neither the physician nor patient need feel demeaned, neglected nor deprived. Both might come away richer and softer for a closer understanding of the complexity of life.

It is our conviction that too many failures in collaboration find their cause in the premature, casual, imprecise labeling of individualistic or unconventional patients as "obstructive" or worse, "noncompliant." Patients nonetheless who "consciously choose not to comply with their physician's prescriptions because they question his judgment, because they believe, rightly or wrongly, that the protocol he has recommended is too radical, or alternatively, too conservative, would not, strictly speaking, be described as noncompliant."[2] Yet negatively perceived patients, regardless of diagnostic accuracy, easily become entrenched in adversarial relationships with those caretakers they most depend upon. Unlike the artist, whose interest it may serve to challenge "the system" and whose success draws upon his individuality, let the patient beware who stretches the norm, however unwittingly, and asks a medical bureaucracy to bend in ways it is unused—or biased against—doing. Such a patient or family incurs the quick approbation of medical staff and risks exclusion from the collaborative process which depends so much for its success on their participation.

In the case of the elderly, failures in collaboration assume a particular poignancy and a more serious urgency. If the aged in our youth-oriented culture already endure a process—not always biologically determined—of diminishing narcissistic replenishment through social isolation, family dispersal, limited mobility, forced retirement, and fixed income, then the misunderstood, sick elderly suffer a triple burden. We postulate that the elderly are particularly vulnerable to negative staff responses not only because of the conscious and unconscious anxiety that chronic or grave illness provokes in all of us—even the initiated doctors and nurses—but because medical economics today presses medical staff into rapid, often sterotyped determinations of prognosis and plan.

We hope to show here that the social worker occupies a position of pivotal influence in a multidisciplinary setting to free patients and staff from such incorrect categorizing in order to achieve creative patient care and staff learning. This same process yields a bonus: the quicker recognition of the truly noncompliant patient and his treatment as a discretely different behavior phenomenon.

Most of the issues raised above find voice in the case example of Mrs. W., a black clinic patient who because of her illness could never very actively participate with staff but depended upon her family to endorse her wishes. This elderly patient was notable for her capacity to surprise, provoke, question, resist, and ultimately—despite initial opposition— achieve staff conversion (compliance!) to her own philosophy. We think she informs us importantly about the elderly by the variety of interventions she prompted from the social worker and which the following presentation will illustrate. This paper relies on one case because it is rich in patient, family and medical community's investment at a most critical time. It could be argued that all cases are not so varied, but we think the ingredients of this case concerning one elderly woman are universal.

Mrs. W., an 84-year-old black woman from Cuba, was brought to the emergency room by her two daughters, Mrs. H. and Mrs. J. She was admitted to an inpatient surgical unit where diagnostic tests during the following week confirmed the presence of a hypernephroma (suspected to be malignant). A positive PAP smear also indicated either cervical or endometrial cancer. Medical records showed that four years prior to admission Mrs. W. had been informed of the same PAP finding but had refused treatment. Medical theory held that Mrs. W.'s present illness was but an advanced (metastatic) stage of the disease diagnosed earlier. Mrs. W. persistently refused surgery over her month-long hospitalization. Despite early family ambivalence and conflict, her family did not feel able to overrule her even in the face of medical pressure. In time, however, after the social worker helped towards an abatement of family disarray, and the medical ear listened more sympathetically to Mrs. W.'s strong and valid preference, the plan changed. Once her condition became stable medically, Mrs. W. was discharged home to her family's care. This plan was augmented by visiting nurse and home health aide services arranged by the worker.

From the beginning, the social worker perceived this situation as likely to require considerable collaborative effort because of the nature of Mrs. W.'s clear refusal of surgery, her family's initial internal discord and the medical staff's difficulty tolerating such "opposition" to their professional recommendation. In what, then, did Mrs. W.'s rebellion reside that she was able to accept partial medical assistance but refuse surgery? The answer lies in the social worker's discovery and assessment of the dynamics that conditioned this deportment through ongoing contact with patient and family.

Case Example

Mrs. W.'s physically ample and soft form, diminutive voice and generally gentle disposition contrasted dramatically with her stubborn determination to have things her way. Though terminally ill, confined to bed, weakened by pain, and infrequently awake, Mrs. W. managed occasionally to smile at a compliment or at a memory. She frequently made withering asides about her doctors who asked her to sign her "death warrant" as she called the surgical consent form. She responded mostly to the touch of comforting hands and her eyes returned her appreciation even if she could not always speak. She seemed at ease accepting help, though with an increasing mixture of wonder and dismay that she was still worth all the fuss.

Mrs. W. was born and raised in Cuba. Widowed in her 40s, she worked as a housekeeper and independently raised seven children and numerous grandchildren. By the time Castro assumed political control, Mrs. W., already in her 60s, had managed with enormous self-confidence to emigrate to Jamaica with five of her children "to be free." Two children remained behind, two settled with her in Jamaica, and three came to the United States. Seven years prior to Mrs. W.'s hospitalization, she permitted Mrs. H. and Mrs. J. to bring her to New York. She had divided her time since arriving between her daughters' two homes but had made one extensive trip to visit her son, Mr. E. in California. Until she had more recently become eligible for SSI and Medicaid, her daughters and son had shared financial responsibility for her.

Mrs. W. had become primarily homebound by increasing infirmity and illness over the previous four years. Undaunted, she had solved this dilemma of reduced mobility (not influence!) by bringing the world to her: children and grandchildren far away wrote and phoned. She augmented their reports by television, radio, magazines and books which she enjoyed best, next to her Bible. Even her priest's affection for her prompted monthly home visits.

Psychosocial Assessment

When Mrs. W. entered the hospital, she brought with her a constellation of beliefs significantly antithetical to those of a medical community. Although she wanted to know what the doctors found, she did not necessarily feel able to follow all of the medical recommendations. Mrs. W., for example, felt capable of relinquishing her full life without prolonging it through the medical technology of modern surgery. She had consistently believed that at her age surgery for cancer would be agonizing and probably palliative at its best. In fact certain research has shown that older patients have an apparent preference for less risk-taking or discomfort rather than for longer life.[3] Since medical staff promised little in terms of length or quality of life post-surgery, she preferred, being devoutly Catholic, to "let God decide when to take me" without, "interfering with His schedule." She had also maintained a high degree of investment in dying with her body outwardly intact, which had less to do with vanity than with a profound belief in the sanctity of life *and* death as natural processes and possibly a belief in the resurrection of the body. It had also to do with her cultural milieu's commitment to individualism, and the fact that in her exalted position as matriarch she was granted particular authority.

The elder daughter, Mrs. H., graced by an assurance that she had been well loved by her mother, could mourn her dying with more grief than anxiety. This deep truth also allowed her to hear, evaluate, and judge options for her mother's care with more realism than resistance. She sometimes rationalized her preferred position by claiming "sole right" to make final decisions on the basis of currently being her mother's primary caretaker. She had promised her mother that under no circumstances would she ever allow surgical intervention and the promise was already four years old.

To Mrs. J. who ran a close second in daily involvement, Mrs. H.'s attitude on "right" was a source of historical and continuing sorrow, frustration, and conflict. Her unresolved struggle for her mother's attention and approval was powerfully rekindled by the illness yet it explained her ability to defer to her mother's and sister's decision.

Mr. E., from California, whom the social worker met only briefly during the earliest phase of hospitalization, was the sole family member with unqualified trust in doctors. Living so far away had precluded closeness with his mother and made him feel angry but unable to claim equal authority with his sisters in making decisions for her care. While he and his sisters initially disagreed vehemently as to the medical recommendation for surgery, they were culturally bound in common devotion to their mother. They considered her the ultimate source of love and authority, truly the axle of her family's wheel.

Interventions

Collaborative effort proceeded through time of admission and full diagnosis; refusal of surgery and transfer to a non-surgical unit for recovery of medical stability; organization and implementation of a satisfactory discharge plan.

Upon admission, Mrs. W. was designated a "high risk" patient. This mandated a social worker's prompt entry and assessment of the need to provide future psychological help and/or concrete services during what is often a wrenching and chaotic hospital experience. During the diagnostic phase the social worker spent time with Mrs. W. exploring her feelings about illness, hospitalization and her attitude specifically towards surgery. By obtaining a full psychosocial history she was able to validate Mrs. W.'s competence. It was the worker's early entry that permitted such thorough understanding and lively engagement of staff.

In the case described, the social worker based delivery of service to Mrs. W. and her family in the belief that an individual has the right to self-determination provided he has knowledge upon which to make his choices and the likely consequences of those choices. This happily coincided with Mrs. W.'s own social milieu's commitment to individualism. Whenever Mrs. W. was available, she was encouraged to maintain her self-confidence since it was obvious that she needed help within the hospital community resisting initial medical bias.

Mrs. W.'s children needed help to say good-bye to their mother, particularly without guilt or recrimination in the event they were to decide to overrule her. The social worker was always a constant sounding board for their thoughts and feelings. This permitted family relationships to continue in a positive way during the stressful terminal period of their mother's illness. This was never truer than initially when sisters and brother were in such sharp and loud disagreement. Efforts were made for each person to leave the other appreciated and intact. Because they were reluctant to leave Mrs. W. during this crisis, the social worker accommodated to their need for informality. She saw them variously around their mother's bedside, in private places claimed from public pathways, or maintained contact through many phone calls. The social worker was a liaison between family and medical staff when direct meetings between these two were difficult to achieve. The social worker spurred the family's careful consideration of all alternatives for treatment and the consequences of their choices.

Mrs. W.'s primary source of joy and comfort was her family. The social worker drew upon their collective sense of responsibility and strength to sustain her with their visits and phone calls. The Cuban and Jamaican embassies were even invoked by the social worker to permit exit visas for her other children so they might see their mother before she died. Her priest was encouraged to visit her regularly in the hospital though it was a long and tiring trip for him to make.

In terms of the hospital community, the social worker tried for the following interventions: she illuminated medical staff of the social milieu in which Mrs. W. was embedded. There was always the hope that by individualizing Mrs. W. the medical staff might modify or abandon their pressure for surgery. Particularly with this older patient whose life had held so many satisfactions, it was important for doctors to understand that her decision was based more on resolve than panic. "A knowledge of the way in which people perceive themselves in relation to their experiences in life and their sense of satisfaction and accomplishment is essential for understanding them as they strive for closure."[4] Such insights helped the physicians later to abandon their initial recommendation without a sense of defeat or failure. With extended knowledge they learned that by allowing Mrs. W. to die in her own way, they were helping her to live in the best way. Once Mrs. W. was transferred to a new floor, the social worker, as the only consistent caretaker, alerted the new medical team there to the likely effects their own disapproval of her refusal for surgery could have e.g., stigmatization, isolation, and psychological abandonment. By exploring with medical staff the motive behind her decision and their responses to them, Mrs. W. achieved their more generous understanding. Additionally, the social worker helped the family to understand the administration's motive behind Mrs. W.'s transfer to a medical floor and ultimate discharge home. By explaining to the family how an acute care hospital is in constant need of free beds, any anxiety the family may have felt that the moves were punitive in nature was removed. It also permited the family to make quicker and more trusting relationships with the new staff members.

Lest the reader conclude a flawless relationship between the social worker and medical staff, there were occasions when the worker herself absorbed or provoked their impatience or anger for her advocacy. Such flare-ups required time and professional discipline to overcome. Interestingly, the social worker also reduced conflicts within the medical community itself. Treatment refusal by competent patients can result in heated debate particularly when "refusal is linked to life-preserving treatments such as . . . surgery."[5] These debates were most visible when socially oriented younger doctors and nurses challenged senior staff who nonetheless were burdened by ultimate case management. Whenever possible, the social worker encouraged those who were most sympathetic to Mrs. W. to spend time with her and her family. By doing so the physicians better understood the impact of illness and treatment refusal on adult children as well as on Mrs. W. Conversely, the worker helped the family to appreciate the complexities of a physician's responsibility and historical bias. She also helped the family separate their more personal struggles from their mothers's.

Lastly, as far as we know, one of the most critical features not usually defined or even acknowledged as a collaborative intervention is the worker's steady self-examination. Though an internal process, its intent is always towards the best use of self with others. Vigilance of one's own feelings and prejudices (sometimes shifting under pressures of time, others' personalities and one's own vagueries), enables the social worker to avoid stereotypical responses. In a medical setting it is noteworthy that the social worker is the only professional normally required to carry such heavy responsibility for introspection in behalf of patient and staff. While training for this is arduous and preoccupying, it is also a source of the worker's success and wisdom.

Summary

It is no longer appropriate in an acute care hospital to await the physician's invitation to serve the elderly patient. The extremity of illness in the elderly knocks on the door of Time, alerting all that the solution this time may be the crucial, if not the final, decision of a patient's life. The complexities of medical care and the newer insights into the social and psychological dynamics of health maintenance makes it necessary for someone to undertake at once the organization of the often conflicting consequences that otherwise interrupt helpful service. Add to this the recognition of honoring a patient's right to choose, in addition to the physician's duty to preserve life, and you have a herculean agenda for a social worker's engagement.

A case was presented here of an 84-year-old woman, incurably ill, whose refusal of surgery was seen at first as a defiance of medical wisdom. For her, as well as for many elderly patients, the technology of modern surgery could promise little in terms of prolongation or improved quality of life. The offer of invasive treatment, though perhaps faithful to strict surgical precepts, failed to achieve a full match of plan to person. Since older person comprise an ever growing percentage of inpatient populations, the risk is great that they will become stereotyped according to a class of patient rather than individualized as their needs actually dictate. In the case discussed, the social worker's activity was preempted by just such an occurrence—the quick and imprecise labeling of an individualistic woman by medical staff hard pressed for time and hindered by economic pressures to classify, treat, and discharge.

The social work interventions in behalf of individualizing and humanizing this elderly patient to professional staff—in our view the cornerstone of comprehensive medical treatment—rested on a combination of the following factors.

1. A recognition that collaborative practice in an acute care setting is hard to achieve but that collective responsibility and accountability is desirable for all. The concept of collaboration was enhanced by the inclusion of patient and family as equal participants with professional staff in the process.
2. A value base which included a belief in the individual's right to self-determination and a respect for the physician's own strict code of ethics.
3. A knowledge of individual psychodynamics and sociocultural influences that permitted this individual woman and her family to withstand the stress of terminal illness, hospitalization, and staff not always sympathetic to her decision to refuse surgery.
4. A rigorous awareness of the social worker's own self in relation to patient, family and staff. By means of a helpful neutrality, the social worker gained the confidence of all participants and permitted each to maintain or achieve a solution of dignity and professional integrity.

REFERENCES

1. Swift, Jonathan. *Polite Conversation In Three Dialogues*, ed. Eric Partridge, Andre Deutsch Ltd., London, 1963, p. 145.

2. Strain, James, J., MD. *Psychological Interventions in Medical Practice*, Appleton-Century-Crofts, New York, 1978, p. 91.

3. Libow, Leslie S., MD. "Care of Elderly: Interface of Clinical and Ethical Decisions," *New York State Journal of Medicine*, December 1981, p. 1900.

4. Monk, Abraham. "Social Work with the Aged: Principles of Practice," *Social Work*, Volume 26, Number 1, January, 1981, p. 91.

5. Libow, Leslie S., MD. *Op.cit.*, p. 1898.

Chapter 11

RESIDENT COUNCILS AND SOCIAL ACTION

Jessica Getzel

Goffman, in his discussion of the asylum, notes how the total institution must encourage dependency in inmates which serves to protect them from each other and the outside world.[1] In any total institution such as a nursing home, the activist quality of a lifetime may fall away for the aged. Even the otherwise defiant and challenging person may become desperate out of her/his dependency for care as personal power ebbs.

One effort at empowering residents of nursing homes that has gained current favor is the Resident Council, a model of democracy superimposed on a hierarchical structure of a custodial institution. This paper will examine the ideals of the Resident Council and the realities of its implementation, as well as the effect on the nursing home milieu. The emerging professional literature on Resident Councils will be reviewed. The social work role in the development and evolution of the Resident Council will be described with particular attention given to the potential conflict between activating residents versus coopting them in the exclusive interest of the organization.

Relevant Literature

Barbara Silverstone sees the function of the nursing home Resident Council as "serve[ing] as a vehicle for residents to exercise their rights and protect their interests by participating fully in the decisions and tasks which affect their everyday lives, both in the home and the outside community."[2] Silverstone makes some useful recommendations about the organization and the function of Resident Councils. An optimistic outlook for Resident Councils is shared by articles on the subject.[3] Resident Councils are seen to have a monitoring function and a therapeutic potential.[4] Some states have built-in requirements for Resident Councils into nursing home regulations. Resident Councils may be seen as an extension of civil rights protection to institutional environment. Miller and Solomon question the extent to which residents can have free expression, if they are dependent on staff in so many intimate ways, including the ongoing running of the Resident Council.[5]

Devitt and Checkoway researched the efficacy of Resident Councils in Illinois prior to being mandated by the state regulations. They found that Resident Councils tended to be founded by administration and staff with little involvement of the residents themselves. Elections of resident members are a recurrent problem and the choice of participants may be determined by administration. Different arrangements for officers appear prevalent from the extremes of no officers, all resident officers, to a mixture of staff, administration and resident officers. Findings indicate a strong dominance of administration. An area of concern is what is the proper role of staff and administration, and could more residents be involved in significant areas of institutional life concerns.[6]

A Proposed Model

Working with a Resident Council requires differential and flexible skills and strategies over a period of time. Without administration's sanction and encouragement, the development of a Resident Council can be an exercise in frustration and futility for staff, and most importantly for the residents who have limited energy to devote to a charade. Resident Councils, if effective, open areas of difficulty and pain. Unless the staff and administration are prepared to give maximum autonomy to a group of elected "volunteer" resident officers and floor captains, they will only add to residents' actual and perceived dependency on the institution.

Not the least able, but the most professional skilled staff should work with residents in the Council. This is not a good experience for new staff but should be seen as a very challenging assignment for a social worker with demonstrable regard for residents and vice versa. The success of a Resident Council rests on two grounds. First, the Council can accomplish some perceivable gains *from* staff and administration which enhances residents' well-being and when they cannot achieve their goals, they are still treated with respect. Secondly, social work skills with membership of a Resident Council should aid with crises of aging which occur, so that members' dignity is maintained.

The introduction of a Resident Council may initially meet with superficial acceptance by both staff and residents. Administration must carefully interpret the function of the Council and emphasize that it is to be a democratic body run by and for the residents. Very often, staff reluctance is an expression of resistance to the explicit demand for resident participation in decision-making and the unconscious recognition of residents as having power over them. Residents may be critical of staff who struggle to do a job, frequently without sufficient recognition. The positive potential is that if the Resident Council is effective, staff will begin to perceive residents as more independent and capable. In addition, the Resident Council can, with encouragement, give positive expression to the good work of staff done on their behalf.

The conceptual approach that has proved useful in work with Resident Councils is the "mediating function" which is an effort to understand and to reconcile needs and resources among residents, staff and administration. Problems arise from routine concerns and periodic crises. William Schwartz sees the mediating function as acknowledging that residents, staff and administration ultimately need one another to do their tasks and that obstacles naturally develop which interfere with symbiotic strivings.[7] In short, administration and staff need residents to fulfill their function; and the extent to which residents respond to their efforts and caring is inextricably tied to a sense of well-being, growth, and belonging. To residents, it is all these things and much more, since their day-to-day living is so dependent on staff and administration.

The success of Resident Councils should be measured by the extent to which real conflicts and concerns are brought out into the open, and different persons in the institution can hear one another and respond honestly to competing claims. This is not done by denying the power of administration or staff but by responsibly sharing decision-making and acknowledging and explaining the "limits" placed on residents' desires for change. The process by its nature is long and arduous, but with professional resolve it is a job worth doing.

The following represents phases in the development of a Resident Council and activities of a social worker serving as a mediating spokesman for the aspirations of very frail and stressed residents in a long-term care facility.

Phase I: The Introduction of the Concept of the Resident Council and Charismatic Leadership

It is not unusual for indigenous leaders among the residents to respond strongly, both positively and negatively, to the introduction of a Resident Council in a nursing home. The worker must recognize natural leaders who develop within the ecological structure of a nursing home (on a floor or section of the facility). The election of officers frequently opens up a contest among residents for prestige and power, two resources in short supply in a nursing home. The worker must carefully open free choice for resident participation and leadership. Frequently a powerful leadership contest may start with active residents joining sides.

An example of the motivation of the charismatic leader is Mrs. G., who had been socially active throughout her life. She believed that residents should participate, otherwise, they would not get the care that they were entitled to. She prided herself on her education and that her husband was a professor. Well-dressed and mannered, Mrs. G. was admired and resented, although this was not expressed directly. Mrs. G felt that residents should be treated well since most residents were the peers of the professional staff. She was willing to serve and made it clear from the start the *she* had distinct views on long-term care. Mrs. G. and other residents needed staff encouragement to risk participation. An unavowed concern was residents' fear that they would antagonize staff. The worker should reach for these concerns. Their anxiety may be expressed in the concern that they cannot adequately represent residents on their floors.

Phase II: Formalization of Structure

A Council structure should be clearly developed and interpreted to residents. It is important to allow Council members to dip into their own organizational experience and have the time so that they can make decisions. This is vital. Resident members often have experience in organizations such as Womens' Clubs, charities, business and labor unions. An attitude of "sharing power" among residents is encouraged as residents are able to discuss their past experiences in kindred organizations. Sharing responsibilities gives recognition to the possibility of the illness and incapacitation of a particular member. An unavowed fear that pervades the group process is the illness or death of a member or a particular leader of the Council. The use of alternates extends membership roles and deals with the problem initially.

Phase III: Engagement of Isolated Residents

The relationship with administrators is crucial in winning broad resident interest in the Council. Regular weekly or bi-weekly meetings are necessary. Administrators should be invited as advisors rather than the powerful adversary.

It is also important to allow structure to arise from resident felt-needs than other short-term considerations. Floors with less functional members may address their concerns more fully by a special subcommittee structure with less formal requirements than a Roberts' Rules format and sub-committees report to the larger Resident Council.

Council members may initially deal with building or institution-wide problems rather than problems with a personalized quality. An effective tool is the use of an "educational seminar" held briefly at the beginning of meetings. It is very helpful to the less functioning member. As the Council grows, less educational seminars may be needed.

Phase IV: Problem-Solving and Felt Concerns

Early issues tend to solidify residents' relationships with one another and underline their need to speak communally and not individually.

For example, new elevators that close too quickly can mobilize Council members who are fearful they may break their hips. The consequence may be planful action. Members ask for incidents of reports from other residents and compile a list of those residents who have not been able to handle elevator doors. In floor meetings residents are helped to report dangerous incidents. A report is written and given to administrators, and an elevator operator replaces manual operation. A small victory, perhaps, but one with considerable meaning to older people who feel they are losing their competence in the environment.

Phase V: Engagement of Key Institutional Personnel

Ongoing effectiveness of Resident Councils rest on their continuing ability to relate to administrative personnel of the nursing home. A worker should help residents explore priorities and develop a Council structure to investigate and report on areas of concern. A structure with medical, nursing and other committees, for example, allows more able residents to participate and do work for Council meetings. Different staff members consult with committees which has the latent function of winning support for the Resident Council from staff and expanding residents' acquaintance with staff and administration.

It is not unusual for the Council to take on the style of the nursing home administration. Residents, with staff support, write their own memos and reports, and have regular appointments with the administration. Consistent relationship with staff must be recognized as more productive than sudden, inflamed encounters with administration when matters get out of hand. Establishing regular meetings with department heads and committee members contribute to the exchange of information but also gives an opportunity for policy to be interpreted by both parties.

A medical committee can investigate crowding in the clinic. Resident observers in the Clinic note conditions and make recommendations to the medical director and nursing director. They request a written response in ten days. Meetings with directors can be fruitful, if residents and their consultants are able to compose complete and precise recommendations. The reports and minutes of the Council are a record for State evaluations of the nursing home.

Phase VI: Enhancement of Resident Solidarity

It is not unusual for residents in the Council leadership to create a sense of closeness. Frequent interaction and the progressive sharing of plans increases socialization. To the extent membership in the Council is open, it may also have a more salutory influence in the institution itself. Evidences of this phase may be seen when members talk more frequently, exchange visits, and share snacks.

Phase VII: Support and Mutual Aid during Membership Crises

Regardless of how competent and accomplished members of the Resident Council may be, the Council must deal with the trauma of the loss of leadership from illness and death. The aging process does not stop. Counselling by social workers allows residents to compensate for functional disabilities. Honest discussion with residents about limitations is vital. Strategic intervention with members with memory loss may permit continued participation despite persistent difficulties. The discomfort members express when a leader of the Council can no longer function necessitates careful and sensitive discussion. In the event of a death of a key member, members must be allowed to grieve ritually and openly in the Council meeting. For example, When Mrs. G., the first president of the Resident Council, died, both staff and residents went to the funeral. Openness about the membership crises and group reactions stimulate renewed commitment to work on the Council by members and staff.

Phase VIII: Community Linkages and Social Action

As the structure and group identification of Resident Council takes mature form, opportunities to link residents activities to their families and outside community groups should take place. One of the most exciting possibilities is coalitions of resident councils in long-term care facilities for the aged. In New York State, the Coalition of Institutionalized Aged and Disabled has worked with the well aged and disabled to increase spending money allowances, leaves of absence for vacations, and increased bed retention periods for those in long-term care. Contact with outside groups legitimizes the considerable activities of the Resident Council and contributes to the community's understanding of the "hidden" aged. Incapacitated aged persons asking for benefits can be very persuasive to state legislators. Families should be kept appraised of the activities of the Resident Council and should be encouraged to use it. Allowances might be made for family or close friends to observe Resident Council meetings on a periodic basis.

Conclusion

Resident Councils can be a significant enhancement function in a nursing home or an empty exercise in futility. Resident participation entails a considerable expenditure of staff efforts and imagination. If the lives of residents are enriched and areas of concern lightened, then it is surely worth the effort for residents, administration, and staff. An honest approach to Resident Councils opens the opportunity for expanded activities despite the aged's frailty and limited mobility. Faith in a human being's capacity for democratic participation and growth should not end when she or he enters a nursing home.

REFERENCES

1. Goffman, Erving. *Asylums* New York: Doubleday, 1961.
2. Silverstone, Barbara. *Establishing Resident Councils*, New York: Federation of Protestant Welfare Agencies, Division of Aging, December 1974, p. 8.
3. Devitt, Mary & Checkoway, Barry. "Participation in Nursing Home Resident Councils: Promise and Practice", *Gerontologist* 22:1, February 1982.
4. *Ibid.*
5. Miller, Irving & Solomon, Renee. "The Development of Group Services for the Elderly," in Carel B. Germain, Editor, *Social Work Practice: People and Environments*, New York, Columbia University Press, 1979, p.p. 90-91.
6. Devitt & Checkoway, *op. cit.*
7. Schwartz, William. "The Social Worker in the Group," *The Social Welfare Forum, 1961*, New York: Columbia University Press, 1961, p.p. 146-171.

AUTHOR INDEX

Abramson, M. 97,111
Albrecht, G. L. 79
Anisman, H. 126

Becker, E. 2,4
Bengston, V. 96,128-129,144
Berkman, B. 60
Binstock, R. 114,126
Blenkner, M. 85,88,96
Blumenfield, S. 60
Bradley-Rawls, M. 129,133,135,144
Brearley, C. P. 2,4
Brody, E. 1,2,4,33,63,78,96,144,149,154
Butler, R. 60

Caplan, G. 151,154
Cantor, M. 96,128,130,144,149,154
Cath, S. 116,118,126
Checkoway, B. 180,185
Cohen, M. G. 168
Cole, C. 33
Copeland, E. J. 133,145
Cottrell, F. 79
Coulton, C. 57,60

Deterre, E. 96
Devitt, M. 180,185
Dobrof, R. 83,84,85-86,95,96,140,145
Dowd, J. 128-129,144
Downing, R. A. 133,145

Eisdorfer, C. 114,126
Engel, G. L. 60
Eribes, R. A. 129,133,135,144
Erickson, E. 38,60,93,96

Fortinsky, R. H. 79
Fulchon, C. 154

Germaine, C. B. 33
Getzel, G. 96

Gitterman, A. 33
Goffman, E. 98,179,185
Golan, N. 78
Goldfarb, A. 33
Granger, C. V. 64,72,78
Greengross, S. 33
Greer, D. S. 79
Gross-Andrews, S. 154
Gustafson, E. 158,168
Guttman, D. 119,126

Hagestad, G. 126
Hamilton, B. B. 79
Hollis, F. 73,79
Horowitz, A. 96
Hubbard, R. W. 79
Hudis, I. 154-155
Huyck, M. D. 79

Jenkins, S. 137,140,145

Kastenbaum, R. 60
Knowles, J. H. 36,60
Koff, T. H. 159,168
Kohl, M. 111
Kohut, H. 117,126
Kostick, A. 168
Kropotkin, P. 151,154
Kurtz, J. J. 168
Kyle, D. G. 168

Levenson, J. 158,162,168
Lewis, H. 111
Libow, L. 60,178
Lieberman, M. 87,89,96
Liton, J. 33
Litwak, E. 96
Lowy, L. 2,3,4

Maddox, G. 60,126
Mahler, M. 118

SUBJECT INDEX

abuse and neglect, in community 26;
  in nursing home 30-31,98,107
aged
  demographics 84,128-130,167
  direct practice 14-17,45-47,50-51,53,
    71-79,87,91,125,174,184
  impact of illness 9-10,102,115-123
  incidence of illness 39,61,113-116
  staff attitudes 37,39,40,56-57,170-171
aging process 10-11,170-171
  chronic illness 102,113
  intervention 9,87,119,122,123-125
  physiological changes 113-114
Alzheimer's disease
  See senile dementia
assessment 11-13,123-124
  in day care 159,162
  with family 150,160
  in hospital 41-45
  in nursing home 142
  in rehabilitation center 62-65,73-75
auxiliary function model 10-33
  description 10-11
  priorities setting 30-31

case management 24-25,104,176
case planning 13-14
  with informal supports 14,144,150,169
community services 8,19-22,23-24,53,65,
    69,73-75,125,132,158,166
  day care 157-168
  home care 22-23,24,72
crisis model 66,85-95
  intervention strategies 66-68,87-89,92,
    94,95

day care 157-168
  characteristics of clients 159
  family intervention 160, 165-167
  groups in 164; institutional linkage 159

intake and referral 159-160
  legislation 167
  mutual aid 164-165
  as respite 8,23,53-54,166-167
  social work function 159,160,162
death and dying 40,85,92-93,94-95,100,
    111,115,173,184
  suicide 101,110
direct practice
  with aged 14-17,45-47,50-51,53,71-79,
    87,91,125,184
  with family 18-19,47-51,53-56,71-79,
    87,88-89,91-92,93-94,150-151
  with groups 17-18,89,91,151-154
discharge planning
  in hospitals 42-45,49-56
  in nursing homes 28-29
  in rehabilitation centers 62,72-77

entitlements 44,51-53,57,151,152,153
  Medicaid 44,51-53,56,57,104-105,135,
    157,158
  Medicare 44,52,57,103,135,157
ethical considerations and values 31,57,
    97-111,125,149-150,170,176,177
  human rights 105-106
  professional codes 103,177
  social justice 108-110
  suicide 101,110
  terminal illness 100,173
  utility 106-107
  virtue 107-108

family
  See also informal supports
  adult day care 8,160,165-167
  hospital 44, 47-51,53-54,169,170
  intervention strategy with 18-19,28,40,
    47-51,53-56,67,71-79,87-89,91-92,
    93-95,124-125,149-154,175

    189

respite care
  day care as 8,23,53-54,166-167
  in the home 19,23,150,151
  need 132

self-help groups 18,75,152-154
senile dementia 53-54,57,109-110
social action 125,152,184-185
  day care legislation 167
social work function

in day care 159,160,162
in hospital 35-60,170-177
in long-term care 7-33,87,88,89,91-92,
  94-95,125
in nursing home 26-28
in rehabilitation center 61-79
with resident councils 30,180,181-182,
  183

volunteers 31,144